THE
STAGE 3
KIDNEY
DISEASE
DIET BOOK

A Kidney Support Cookbook
For Stopping Chronic
Decline in Renal Function

DR. GEORGINA TRACY

The Stage 3 Kidney Disease Diet Book

A Kidney Support Cookbook for Stopping Chronic
Decline in Renal Function

Dr. Georgina Tracy

Disclaimer

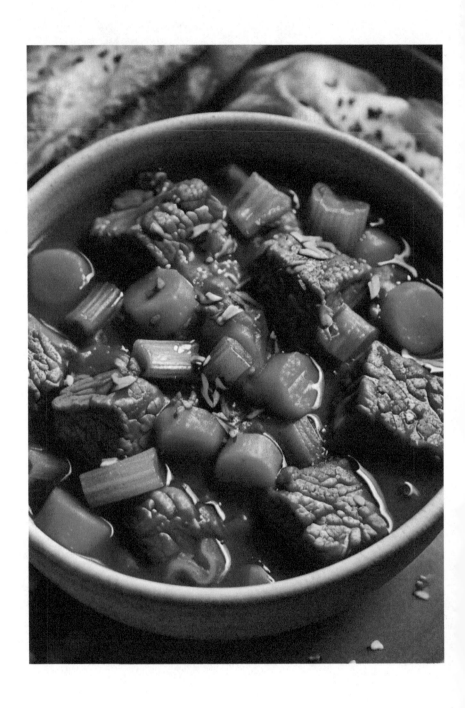

TABLE OF CONTENTS

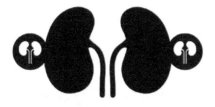

INTRODUCTION

Welcome to the New Edition

Welcome back, and if this is your first time, I'm thrilled to have you here. I'm Dr. Georgina Tracy, and whether you're familiar with the previous edition or this is your first encounter with my work, let me start by saying: you're not alone on this journey.

You see, when I released the first edition of this cookbook, I shared the story of a dear friend of mine, Samuel. At the time, I wrote about his battle with stage 3 kidney disease—how he transformed his lifestyle, fought through the fear and uncertainty, and ultimately became an inspiration to everyone around him. But here's the thing: the Samuel I told you about in that first edition was more than just a man who faced a diagnosis. He was someone I knew well, someone whose struggles hit close to home. And today, I want to tell you the full story.

Why This Cookbook is Different: Focusing on Easy, Practical Solutions

Before I share more about Samuel, let's talk about why this new edition is important. You've likely read other cookbooks that bombard you with technical details and complex medical jargon, but if you've heard all that from your doctor already, you don't need it here, right? What you need are simple, practical solutions—and that's exactly what this book will give you.

In this new edition, I've cut out the fluff and focused on what will actually help you in your day-to-day life. We're talking easy-to-make recipes, meal planning tips, and strategies that you can start using right away. So, let's take this journey together, step by step.

How to Use This Cookbook for Your Stage 3 CKD Journey

This cookbook is designed to guide you through every aspect of managing your kidney health, without overwhelming you. Here's a sneak peek into what you'll find:

✓ Quick Overview of Stage 3 CKD: A simple, no-nonsense refresher on what Stage 3 CKD means and why your diet matters.

✓ Key Dietary Guidelines: We'll keep it practical. Easy guidelines for managing sodium, potassium, and phosphorus levels without overcomplicating things.

✓ Easy, Delicious Recipes: From breakfast to dinner, and everything in between, I've got you covered with meals that are both kidney-friendly and flavorful.

✓ Meal Planning and Beyond: Planning your meals shouldn't be a chore. I'll help you set up a routine with a 7-day meal plan and tips that make it all manageable.

✓ Bonus Resources: I'm giving you access to printable tools—meal planners, grocery checklists, and cheat sheets that will keep you organized and stress-free.

Revisiting Samuel's Story

Now, let's get back to Samuel. When I first shared his story, I talked about how he was a high school teacher, a dedicated family man, and how his diagnosis of Stage 3 kidney disease flipped his world upside down. But what I didn't tell you was how dire things really were for him at the time.

Samuel wasn't just a man who liked to cook for his family; he was the kind of guy who poured everything into his job and his home life, often forgetting to take care of himself. By the time he came to me, his kidney function had already dropped to a scary 39%. I remember the day he walked into my office. He didn't come with just lab results—he came with a deep, unspoken fear. His father had passed away from complications due to kidney failure, and Samuel couldn't shake the feeling that he was heading down the same path.

But here's what really shocked me—and him. When we dove into his diet and lifestyle, it became clear that Samuel's problem wasn't just about what he ate. It was about how he lived. He was burning the candle at both ends, working late into the night, running on caffeine and processed snacks, and barely getting any sleep. His body was telling him to slow down, but Samuel, being the tough and driven man he was, kept pushing.

The turning point came during a family vacation. It was supposed to be a relaxing trip, but Samuel collapsed from exhaustion while they were out hiking. That's when he realized he couldn't ignore his health anymore. His kids, who were just teenagers at the time, were scared out of their minds. His wife, Em, stood over him in tears. That was the moment he decided things had to change—for good.

When Samuel started making those changes, it wasn't just about swapping out junk food for veggies. He had to reevaluate everything: how he balanced his life, how he handled stress, and how he prioritized his health. And yes, there were setbacks. He struggled to stick with it at first, but the more he pushed forward, the more he realized that taking care of his kidneys wasn't just about staying alive—it was about truly living.

Today, Samuel's kidney function is, on average, stable at 47%—and has shown potential for getting even better, and he's not just surviving—he's thriving. He still teaches, but he makes time for himself and his family. He even leads workshops for other teachers dealing with chronic illness, showing them how they, too, can reclaim their health. And the best part? He's watching his kids grow up, something he once feared he'd miss.

Your story could be next!

Look, Samuel's journey isn't just inspiring—it's a reminder that no matter where you are right now, you can make a change. You don't have to have all the answers today, and you don't have to do it alone. This book is here to guide you, just like I was there for Samuel. Together, we'll make the small, powerful changes that can make all the difference.

So, let's get started.

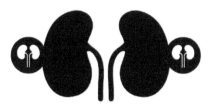

CHAPTER 1: QUICK OVERVIEW OF STAGE 3 CKD

What You Really Need to Know About Stage 3a and 3b CKD

Okay, so you've been told you have Stage 3 CKD. I know that hearing the words Stage 3 can sound scary, but let's take a deep breath and break it down. Stage 3 CKD is split into two parts: Stage 3a and Stage 3b. The main difference between them? The level of kidney function, which is measured by something called your glomerular filtration rate, or GFR for short.

Here's what it means in plain language:

Stage 3a: Your GFR is between 45 and 59. This means your kidneys are working at about half their full capacity. You might not feel any symptoms yet, or you could have some mild ones like fatigue or changes in urination.

Stage 3b: Your GFR is between 30 and 44. At this stage, your kidneys are struggling a bit more, and you might start noticing symptoms like swelling in your hands or feet, or more frequent trips to the bathroom.

Now, let me reassure you: **Stage 3 is manageable.** Your kidneys are still doing their job, even though they need a little help. This is where you come in! By making some key changes to your diet and lifestyle, you can slow down the progression of the disease and give your kidneys the best chance at staying strong for as long as possible.

But here's the deal—every person is different, so while your GFR number gives us an idea of your kidney health, it's not the whole picture. What's important is how you feel, how your body responds, and what you do moving forward. And that's where we'll focus next.

The Role of Diet in Slowing Disease Progression (In Simple Terms)

I know you've probably heard this before, but it's worth repeating: **what you eat matters**—a lot! When it comes to CKD, your kidneys are like a filter for everything you consume. The less work they have to do, the better they function over time. So, we want to give your kidneys a bit of a break by being mindful of certain things, like sodium, potassium, phosphorus, and protein.

Here's what that looks like, in simple terms:

✓ Sodium (Salt): Too much sodium makes your kidneys work harder, and it can cause your body to hold onto extra water, leading to swelling and high blood pressure. By cutting down on salt, you're doing your kidneys a huge favor. Trust me, your body will thank you for it.

✓ Potassium: This mineral is tricky because your body needs it, but too much can be harmful to your kidneys. Certain foods are high in potassium, so it's important to know what to eat and what to avoid. Don't worry, I'll show you some delicious low-potassium options in the recipes!

✓ Phosphorus: Phosphorus is another mineral that can build up in your blood if your kidneys aren't filtering properly. When this happens, it can weaken your bones and affect your heart. By watching your phosphorus intake, you're helping keep everything in balance.

✓ Protein: Now, this one is a bit more personal. Your body needs protein to stay strong, but eating too much can put extra strain on your kidneys. The key is finding the right amount for your body. In this book, I've got plenty of recipes that strike a balance, so you're still getting enough protein without overdoing it.

That's it! Nothing too complicated—just a few simple shifts that can make a world of difference for your kidneys. Remember, it's not about perfection. It's about making consistent, small changes that will add up over time.

So, as we move forward, we'll focus on those key areas to help keep your kidneys in good shape. I'm here to guide you every step of the way, and by the end of this, you'll feel empowered and ready to take control of your health.

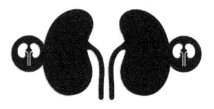

CHAPTER 2: JUMPSTART TO KIDNEY-FRIENDLY EATING

The 5 Most Important Dietary Changes You Can Make Today

Ready to jumpstart your kidney-friendly eating? Don't worry, you don't need to overhaul your entire diet in one day. The key here is small, manageable changes that can make a big impact over time. Here are the five most important dietary changes you can start making right now:

Cut Back on Sodium

Sodium, or salt, is everywhere, but for your kidneys' sake, we need to dial it back. Aim to cook with less salt and reach for herbs, spices, and other flavor boosters instead. Trust me, once you get used to it, you won't miss that extra salt at all!

Watch Your Protein Intake

Your body needs protein, but with CKD, it's all about balance. Too much can strain your kidneys, so we want to get just the right amount. The recipes in this book will help you find that sweet spot without compromising taste.

Limit Processed Foods

Processed foods are sneaky—they're often loaded with sodium, phosphorus, and potassium. Think canned soups, pre-packaged meals, and fast food. Try to swap those out for fresh, whole ingredients whenever you can.

Stay Hydrated (But Not Too Much!)

Water is good, but too much can be tough on your kidneys. Listen to your body and stay hydrated, but don't go overboard. I'll give you some tips later on how to find the right balance.

Keep an Eye on Potassium and Phosphorus

These two minerals are tricky because your kidneys aren't filtering them as well as they used to. High levels can build up and cause problems, so it's important to monitor your intake. Don't worry, I'll guide you on which foods to enjoy and which ones to be mindful of.

These small changes are where you can start, and as you go, they'll feel less like "rules" and more like second nature.

Simple Guidelines for Sodium, Potassium, and Phosphorus Intake

Now, let's break it down a little more. I know it can feel overwhelming when you hear, "Watch your sodium, potassium, and phosphorus," but here's how to think about it in simpler terms:

✓ Sodium: **Aim for less than 1,500 mg per day.** Cutting down on sodium helps reduce swelling and manage blood pressure, both of which are critical for your kidneys. That means skipping the salt shaker and steering clear of highly processed foods like canned soups, snacks, and pre-packaged meals. Don't worry, though—there are plenty of other ways to flavor your meals that I'll show you in this book!

✓ Potassium: For stage 3 CKD, potassium intake is often monitored closely. However, the specific potassium limit varies based on individual needs and lab results. **Generally, potassium intake for stage 3 patients**

should stay between 2,000 and 3,000 mg per day.
Some people may need to aim lower, especially if their
potassium levels are high, but always check with your
healthcare provider to determine the best range for you. In
this book, I'll guide you towards lower-potassium foods
that are still packed with flavor!

✓ Phosphorus: For stage 3 CKD, phosphorus intake should
usually be limited to **800-1,000 mg per day.** Excess
phosphorus can lead to bone and heart problems as it
builds up in your blood, so it's important to be mindful of
foods high in phosphorus like dairy products, processed
foods, and sodas (Especially dark colas). Don't worry—I've
made sure the recipes here are low in phosphorus to help
keep your levels in check.

Simple, right? Just keeping these three things in check will
make a world of difference for your kidneys. You've got this!

Easy Swaps: How to Make Your Favorite Meals Kidney-Friendly

Okay, I know what you're thinking—"But what about my favorite meals?" Don't worry! You don't have to give up the foods you love; you just need to make a few simple swaps to make them kidney-friendly. Here are some quick ideas:

Instead of mashed potatoes, try mashed cauliflower.

You still get that creamy texture without all the potassium!

Instead of salty snacks, go for homemade popcorn with a sprinkle of herbs.

Crunchy, satisfying, and way lower in sodium.

Instead of canned soup, make a quick homemade version.

Use low-sodium broth and fresh veggies—you'll be amazed at how much better it tastes.

Instead of regular pasta sauce, make your own with low-potassium ingredients.

Skip the heavy tomatoes and use a garlic and olive oil base with roasted veggies for flavor.

These are just a few ideas, and you'll find plenty more in the recipes ahead. The point is, you don't have to feel deprived—just get a little creative!

Meal Planning for Beginners

Now, let's talk about meal planning. I know it can seem like a chore, but trust me, it's one of the best things you can do to stay on track with your kidney health. And here's the best part: it doesn't have to be complicated!

Here's how to get started with meal planning:

Pick a day to plan and prep.

Most people find that Sunday works best, but pick whatever day works for you. This is your time to sit down, think about what you want to eat, and get everything ready.

Choose meals that fit your schedule.

Got a busy week? Go for simple, quick meals that don't require a lot of prep. I've included plenty of easy recipes that you can whip up in no time.

Make a shopping list.

Stick to the kidney-friendly ingredients we've talked about. It's easier to stay on track when you've already bought what you need and aren't tempted by unhealthy options.

Prep in batches.

Cook once, eat multiple times. You can make big batches of certain meals, like soups or stews, and freeze them for later. It saves time and keeps you from reaching for something less healthy in a pinch.

Don't be afraid to repeat meals.

It's okay to eat the same meal a couple of times in a week! Find what works for you and stick with it. The more you practice meal planning, the easier it will get.

And guess what? In the next section, I've even included a 7-day meal plan to get you started. It's packed with easy, delicious meals that are perfectly balanced for your kidney health.

I LOOK FORWARD TO HEARING FROM YOU!

WHETHER YOU'VE JUST STARTED COOKING OR YOU'RE ALREADY ENJOYING THE RECIPES, I'D LOVE TO HEAR FROM YOU! YOUR FEEDBACK HELPS ME IMPROVE AND ALSO SUPPORTS OTHERS IN THEIR JOURNEY WITH CKD.

HOW TO LEAVE A REVIEW:

1. SCAN THE QR CODE BELOW WITH YOUR PHONE OR QR CODE SCANNER APP.
2. FOLLOW THE LINK TO THE REVIEW PAGE.
3. GIVE YOUR RATING & SHARE YOUR THOUGHTS!

EVERY REVIEW, NO MATTER HOW BRIEF, MAKES A BIG DIFFERENCE. THANK YOU SO MUCH FOR YOUR SUPPORT!

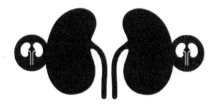

CHAPTER 3: 7-DAY KIDNEY-FRIENDLY MEAL PLAN

We're about to dive into a week-long journey of kidney-friendly eating that's simple, balanced, and delicious. I know how overwhelming meal planning can feel, especially when you're managing something as serious as Stage 3 CKD. But trust me, I've been there with many patients, and I'm here to guide you every step of the way.

This 7-day meal plan is designed to help you feel confident about what's going on your plate, knowing that each meal is carefully curated with your kidney health in mind. We'll break it down day by day, showing you exactly what to eat for breakfast, lunch, dinner, and snacks. And don't worry, I'll even include a complete nutritional breakdown for each day so you know exactly what you're eating—because knowledge is power, right? Let's get started!"

Day-by-Day Menu for Managing Stage 3 CKD

Day 1

- Breakfast: Egg White and Veggie Scramble (with a slice of whole wheat toast)
- Snack: Sliced Apples with Almond Butter
- Lunch: Tuna Salad (low-sodium tuna, light mayo, whole wheat bread) + side of unsalted rice cakes
- Snack: Cucumber Slices with Lemon and Olive Oil
- Dinner: Herb-Roasted Chicken with Quinoa + side of roasted zucchini

Nutritional Info for Day 1: Calories: 1,600 | Protein: 70g | Carbs: 180g | Sodium: 700mg | Cholesterol: 150mg | Potassium: 1,800mg | Phosphorus: 900mg

Day 2

- Breakfast: Low-Sodium Oatmeal with Blueberries
- Snack: Carrot and Cucumber Sticks with Hummus

- Lunch: Quinoa Salad with Cucumbers and Olive Oil Dressing + a side of whole grain crackers
- Snack: Sliced Bell Peppers with Low-Sodium Cream Cheese
- Dinner: Grilled Salmon with Steamed Asparagus + side of brown rice

Nutritional Info for Day 2: Calories: 1,650 | Protein: 75g | Carbs: 170g | Sodium: 750mg | Cholesterol: 120mg | Potassium: 1,700mg | Phosphorus: 950mg

Day 3

- Breakfast: Applesauce Pancakes (low-sodium, no butter)
- Snack: Low-Sodium Rice Crackers with Hummus
- Lunch: Kidney-Friendly Turkey Sandwich (low-sodium turkey, whole wheat bread) + side of carrot sticks
- Snack: Fresh Pear Slices with Almonds
- Dinner: Baked Chicken Thighs with Roasted Carrots + mashed cauliflower

Nutritional Info for Day 3: Calories: 1,680 | Protein: 72g | Carbs: 175g | Sodium: 720mg | Cholesterol: 110mg | Potassium: 1,600mg | Phosphorus: 870mg

Day 4

- Breakfast: Low-Potassium Smoothie Bowl (with berries and almond milk)
- Snack: Unsalted Rice Cakes with Peanut Butter
- Lunch: Lentil Soup (low-sodium broth, kidney-friendly veggies) + whole wheat toast
- Snack: Homemade Low-Sodium Trail Mix (unsalted nuts, dried cranberries)
- Dinner: Turkey Meatballs with Kidney-Safe Tomato Sauce + side of brown rice

Nutritional Info for Day 4: Calories: 1,700 | Protein: 65g | Carbs: 190g | Sodium: 650mg | Cholesterol: 100mg | Potassium: 1,750mg | Phosphorus: 900mg

Day 5

- Breakfast: Chia Seed Pudding (made with almond milk)
- Snack: Air-Popped Popcorn with Olive Oil and Herbs
- Lunch: Grilled Veggie Sandwich with Hummus + side of low-sodium cheese
- Snack: Low-Sodium Cheese and Whole Grain Crackers
- Dinner: Grilled Tilapia with Lemon and Quinoa + steamed broccoli

Nutritional Info for Day 5: Calories: 1,650 | Protein: 68g | Carbs: 180g | Sodium: 670mg | Cholesterol: 90mg | Potassium: 1,720mg | Phosphorus: 880mg

Day 6

- Breakfast: Soft-Boiled Egg Whites on Whole Grain Toast
- Snack: Cucumber Slices with Lemon and Olive Oil
- Lunch: Low-Sodium Chicken Soup with Rice + a slice of whole wheat bread
- Snack: Sliced Apples with Almond Butter
- Dinner: Low-Sodium Beef Stew (with kidney-safe veggies) + mashed potatoes

Nutritional Info for Day 6: Calories: 1,650 | Protein: 70g | Carbs: 170g | Sodium: 680mg | Cholesterol: 95mg | Potassium: 1,740mg | Phosphorus: 880mg

Day 7

- Breakfast: Kidney-Safe Berry Smoothie (using almond milk, strawberries, and blueberries)
- Snack: Low-Sodium Rice Crackers with Hummus

- Lunch: Egg Salad (with egg whites, low-sodium mayo, on whole wheat toast) + sliced cucumbers
- Snack: Fresh Pear Slices with Almonds
- Dinner: Baked Lemon Herb Chicken with Steamed Carrots + brown rice

Nutritional Info for Day 7: Calories: 1,680 | Protein: 68g | Carbs: 180g | Sodium: 660mg | Cholesterol: 85mg | Potassium: 1,750mg | Phosphorus: 870mg

Now that you've had a chance to see a full 7-day meal plan, I bet you're wondering, 'How can I make this work for me on a regular basis?' Well, my dear, I'm going to show you exactly how to take the reins and build your very own meal plans. Here's how we do it:

✓ Start with Breakfast
- Make sure to get some protein in the morning. You could start with egg whites, a kidney-safe smoothie, or even oatmeal with a side of berries.
- Don't be afraid to add some healthy fats like almond butter to boost calories.

✓ Keep Your Lunch Simple but Filling

- Salads with lean proteins like chicken or tuna are great. Add a healthy side, such as quinoa or whole wheat bread, to increase your calorie count.
- Keep dressings light and low in sodium—olive oil and lemon are your friends here!

✓ Balance Your Dinner

- Dinner should be a good balance of lean protein, veggies, and some complex carbohydrates.
- Dishes like grilled salmon with steamed veggies and brown rice or turkey meatballs with low-sodium sauce are perfect for your kidney health.

✓ Snacks Are Key

- Snacks are where you can sneak in extra calories without adding too much sodium or potassium.
- Try unsalted nuts, sliced fruit with almond butter, low-sodium crackers with hummus, or popcorn with olive oil and herbs.

✓ Personalizing Your Plan

- The great thing about having so many options in this cookbook is that you can mix and match meals. Use what you have, and don't be afraid to swap similar ingredients based on availability or preference.
- Just make sure to monitor your sodium, potassium, and phosphorus intake while keeping your calories where you need them to feel full and energetic."

Weekly Shopping List for the Meal Plan

Produce

- 1 bunch fresh parsley
- 1 bunch fresh basil
- 1 bunch fresh dill
- 1 lemon
- 1 cucumber
- 1 zucchini
- 1 head broccoli
- 1 bunch asparagus
- 1 lb carrots
- 1 small pear
- 1 small apple
- 1 small watermelon
- 1 small honeydew melon
- 1 pint blueberries
- 1 pint strawberries
- 1 pint raspberries
- 1 small peach
- 1 bunch spinach
- 1 bunch lettuce (shredded)
- 2 bell peppers (variety of colors)

Protein & Dairy

- 2 chicken breasts
- 2 small salmon fillets
- 2 small tilapia fillets
- 1 lb lean ground turkey
- 1 lb lean ground beef
- 4 large egg whites
- 1/2 lb shrimp
- 1 block firm tofu
- 1 small pork tenderloin
- Low-sodium cheese (2 oz)
- Unsalted almond butter
- Low-sodium cream cheese

Grains & Legumes

- 1/2 cup quinoa
- 1/2 cup brown rice
- 1/2 cup couscous
- 1/4 cup lentils

- 1 loaf whole wheat bread (low sodium)
- 1 package low-sodium whole wheat burger buns
- 8 low-sodium whole grain crackers
- 1 package unsalted rice cakes

Pantry Staples

- 1 jar unsalted peanut butter
- 1 jar unsweetened almond milk
- 1 jar low-sodium hummus
- 1 jar low-sodium mustard
- 1 jar low-sodium tomato sauce
- 1 bottle olive oil
- 1 jar light mayonnaise (low sodium)

- 1 jar low-sodium soy sauce alternative
- 1 container old-fashioned oats
- 1 container low-sodium vegetable broth
- 1 container low-sodium chicken broth
- 1 container low-sodium beef broth

Spices & Condiments

- Ground cinnamon
- Dried thyme
- Dried rosemary
- Garlic powder
- Lemon juice
- Chia seeds (optional)
- Salt-free seasoning (optional)

Alright, now that you've seen what goes into a full week of kidney-friendly meals, let me make your life even easier! Included in this cookbook, you'll find a printable grocery list template. Trust me, it's going to be your new best friend when it comes to staying organized and stress-free while grocery shopping.

You can use this printable list to plan out future meals by grouping ingredients into categories, just like the shopping list you see here. It helps you stay on track and ensures you never forget an ingredient! Whether you're planning another 7-day meal plan or just picking up a few essentials, the printable list will give you the structure to make shopping smooth and efficient. Plus, you can reuse it as many times as you like—just fill it in with the meals and snacks you want for the week, and voilà! You're all set to stay kidney-healthy and organized.

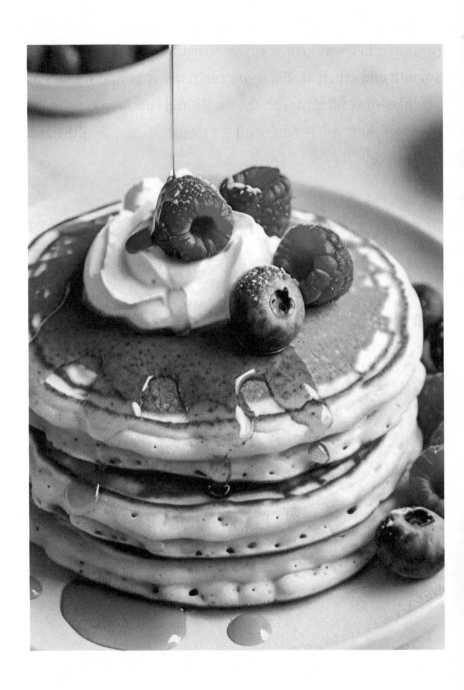

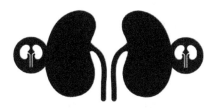

CHAPTER 4: SOURCING AND PREPPING KIDNEY-FRIENDLY INGREDIENTS

When following a kidney-friendly diet, it's important to know exactly what's going into your meals. Some ingredients, like low-sodium turkey or low-potassium vegetables, aren't always easy to find, and preparing them yourself can seem daunting. In this chapter, I'll walk you through the most common ingredients in this cookbook, showing you how to find safe store-bought options and offering simple ways to prepare them at home.

1. Low-Sodium Deli Meats (Turkey, Chicken, etc.)

✓ What to Look For in Stores: When shopping for low-sodium deli meats, check for labels like "low sodium" or "no added salt." Some brands like *Boar's Head Low-Sodium Turkey Breast and Applegate Naturals® No Salt Added Oven Roasted Turkey Breast* offer kidney-friendly options.

✓ **How to Prepare at Home:** If you want more control over sodium levels, you can roast your own turkey breast at home. Simply season with herbs, olive oil, and pepper (avoiding salt), bake until fully cooked, and slice it thinly for sandwiches.

2. Low-Potassium Vegetables

✓ **What to Look For in Stores:** Many fresh vegetables are naturally low in potassium, such as bell peppers, cucumbers, and zucchini. Look for fresh, organic produce whenever possible. When using canned or frozen vegetables, choose brands that are labeled "no added salt."

✓ **How to Prepare at Home:** If you use higher-potassium vegetables like potatoes or carrots, you can lower their potassium content by peeling, chopping, and boiling them in a large pot of water. Drain and rinse the vegetables afterward to further reduce potassium.

3. Low-Sodium Cheese

✓ What to Look For in Stores: For kidney-friendly cheese options, look for "low-sodium" or "reduced sodium" varieties. Brands like *Lucerne Low-Sodium Swiss Cheese or BelGioioso Fresh Mozzarella, No Salt Added* are good options.

✓ How to Prepare at Home: If you're using regular cheese but want to reduce its sodium, you can rinse shredded or sliced cheese briefly in cool water before using it in recipes. This can remove a small portion of the surface sodium.

4. Unsalted Nuts and Seeds

✓ What to Look For in Stores: Opt for raw, unsalted nuts and seeds. Almonds, walnuts, sunflower seeds, and pumpkin seeds are great options. You can find unsalted varieties from brands like *Planters Unsalted Nuts or Simple Truth Organic Unsalted Seeds.*

✓ How to Prepare at Home: If you purchase raw nuts and want a roasted flavor, you can roast them at home without adding salt. Simply spread the nuts on a baking sheet and roast at 350°F for 10-15 minutes, stirring occasionally.

5. Low-Sodium Broths and Sauces

✓ **What to Look For in Stores:** Low-sodium broths are essential for many recipes. Brands like *Swanson® Unsalted Chicken Broth and Pacific Foods Organic Low-Sodium Vegetable Broth* are great options. When buying sauces like tomato or pasta sauce, choose brands that have less than 140mg of sodium per serving.

✓ **How to Prepare at Home:** Making your own broth is easy! Simply simmer vegetables, herbs, and spices (without salt) in water for 1-2 hours. For chicken or beef broth, add bones to the pot and cook over low heat for a richer flavor. Strain and store in the fridge or freezer.

6. Low-Sodium Mustard and Condiments

✓ **What to Look For in Stores:** Look for mustard and other condiments labeled "low sodium" or "no salt added." *Annie's Naturals No-Salt-Added Mustard and Westbrae Natural Unsweetened Ketchup* are great options.

✓ **How to Prepare at Home:** You can make your own mustard by combining mustard powder, water, and vinegar, adding herbs and spices to taste. For ketchup, blend tomatoes with vinegar, garlic, and a touch of honey or sugar, cooking over low heat to thicken.

7. Low-Sodium, Kidney-Friendly Snacks

✓ What to Look For in Stores: Finding kidney-friendly snacks can be tricky. Brands like *Simple Mills Almond Flour Crackers and Mary's Gone Crackers* offer low-sodium, healthy options. You can also look for plain rice cakes, unsalted popcorn, and unsweetened applesauce.

✓ How to Prepare at Home: If you enjoy baking, you can make your own low-sodium crackers using whole grains and seeds. For popcorn, use an air-popper and season with herbs and olive oil instead of butter and salt.

8. Low-Sodium Bread and Whole Grain Products

✓ What to Look For in Stores: Many breads are high in sodium, so it's important to find low-sodium or no-salt-added options. *Food for Life Ezekiel Low Sodium Bread and Alvarado St. Bakery Essential Flax Low Sodium Bread* are great choices.

✓ How to Prepare at Home: Baking your own bread can be a satisfying and kidney-friendly option. Try using whole wheat or spelt flour and avoiding any added salt. There are many simple bread machine recipes that are sodium-free and perfect for sandwiches and toast.

9. Low-Phosphorus Dairy Alternatives (Milk, Yogurt)

✓ **What to Look For in Stores:** Phosphorus can be a concern when it comes to dairy products, so opting for alternatives like unsweetened almond milk, coconut milk, or rice milk is a great idea. Brands like *Silk Unsweetened Almond Milk and So Delicious Coconut Milk* are safe choices. For yogurt, you can choose *Silk Almondmilk Yogurt* or *So Delicious Coconut Yogurt*, which have lower phosphorus than regular dairy.

✓ **How to Prepare at Home:** If you want to make your own dairy alternatives, homemade almond milk is easy to prepare. Simply blend soaked almonds with water, strain through a cheesecloth, and enjoy! For a thicker yogurt alternative, you can ferment almond or coconut milk with a probiotic culture.

10. Low-Sodium Canned Tuna and Fish

✓ **What to Look For in Stores:** Regular canned tuna and fish can be very high in sodium. Look for brands like *Safe Catch Elite Low Sodium Tuna or Wild Planet No Salt Added Wild Albacore Tuna*. For other canned fish options, check the sodium content, or opt for fresh fish when possible.

✓ How to Prepare at Home: If you can't find low-sodium canned tuna, you can poach fresh tuna or other fish at home in water or a low-sodium broth, then store it in the fridge for use in salads and sandwiches. This way, you avoid the high sodium content of pre-packaged options.

11. Low-Sodium Seasoning Alternatives

✓ What to Look For in Stores: Instead of salt-heavy spice blends, look for seasoning mixes that are marked "no salt added" or "low sodium." *Mrs. Dash® Salt-Free Seasoning Blends and Penzeys Spices Salt-Free Seasonings* are great choices for adding flavor without the sodium. You can also find low-sodium soy sauce alternatives like Bragg Liquid Aminos or Coconut Aminos.

✓ How to Prepare at Home: You can make your own seasoning blends at home using fresh herbs, garlic, onion powder, cumin, paprika, and other spices. Avoid store-bought blends that often sneak in sodium under names like "salt" or "sodium chloride."

12. Low-Sodium Nut Butters

✓ **What to Look For in Stores:** Many nut butters, such as peanut butter, can contain added salt. Choose varieties that are labeled "unsalted" or "no added salt." Brands like *Maranatha No Salt Added Almond Butter and Justin's Unsalted Peanut Butter* are excellent kidney-friendly options.

✓ **How to Prepare at Home:** Making your own nut butter is as simple as blending unsalted nuts in a food processor until they reach a smooth, creamy consistency. You can add a little olive oil for smoothness and store it in an airtight jar.

13. Low-Sodium Canned Beans

✓ **What to Look For in Stores:** When buying canned beans, choose brands that offer "no salt added" varieties. *Eden Organic No Salt Added Beans and Westbrae Natural Organic No Salt Added Beans* are great choices. If you can't find these, look for regular canned beans with lower sodium levels and rinse them thoroughly before using.

✓ **How to Prepare at Home:** You can also prepare dried beans at home, which allows you full control over the sodium content. Soak the beans overnight, then cook them in water until tender. You can store them in the fridge or freeze them for later use.

14. Low-Potassium and Low-Phosphorus Flour Alternatives

✓ What to Look For in Stores: For baking, it's important to choose flours that are low in phosphorus and potassium. Whole wheat flour and spelt flour are generally lower in these nutrients than all-purpose flour. Look for brands like *Bob's Red Mill Spelt Flour or Arrowhead Mills Organic Whole Wheat Flour.*

✓ How to Prepare at Home: If you enjoy making your own baked goods, experiment with different flour alternatives that suit your taste and dietary needs. Using spelt flour or a mixture of whole wheat and all-purpose flour can help reduce phosphorus intake while still creating delicious baked goods.

15. Kidney-Friendly Oils and Fats

✓ What to Look For in Stores: Choosing the right oils can make a big difference in your kidney-friendly diet. Olive oil, avocado oil, and flaxseed oil are all great, heart-healthy options. Brands like *California Olive Ranch Extra Virgin*

Olive Oil or Chosen Foods Avocado Oil are excellent for cooking or drizzling on salads.

✓ **How to Prepare at Home:** There's no need to make your own oils, but storing oils properly is important. Keep them in a cool, dark place to preserve their health benefits, and opt for extra virgin varieties when possible, as they retain more nutrients.

16. Low-Sodium, Low-Sugar Jams and Spreads

✓ **What to Look For in Stores:** Many jams and spreads are loaded with sugar and sometimes salt. Look for options labeled "no sugar added" or "low sodium." Brands like *St. Dalfour All Natural Fruit Spread and Polaner All Fruit Spreadable Fruit* offer great alternatives without the added sugars or sodium.

✓ **How to Prepare at Home:** You can make your own low-sugar fruit spread by simmering fresh or frozen berries with a small amount of honey or maple syrup. For a thicker consistency, add a tablespoon of chia seeds to help gel the mixture.

You know, cooking for your kidneys doesn't have to be complicated or overwhelming. It's all about knowing what works for you and making those small, manageable choices. Whether you're grabbing some low-sodium turkey at the store or roasting up your own batch at home, you've got options. This guide is here to help you take the guesswork out of it all, so you can feel confident every time you step into the kitchen.

At the end of the day, what matters most is that you're nourishing your body with foods that not only taste good but also support your kidney health. I've got your back, and together, we're making sure your meals are as delicious as they are kidney-friendly. You're already doing something amazing for your health, and this is just another step in the right direction!

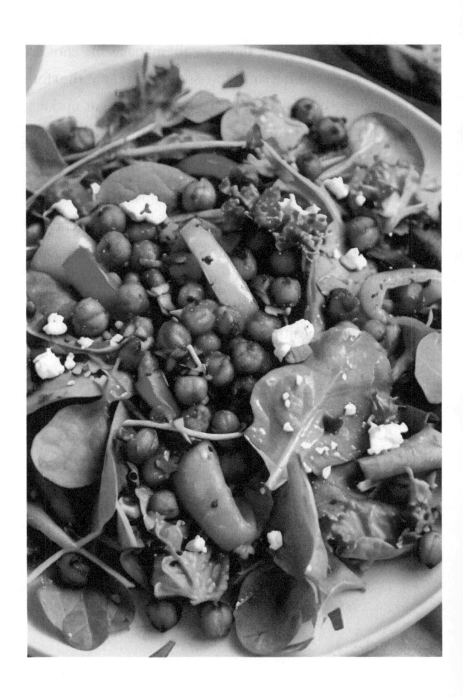

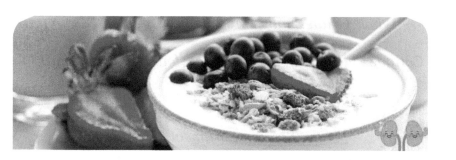

CHAPTER 5: BREAKFAST RECIPES FOR STAGE 3 CKD

Egg White and Veggie Scramble

Low-Sodium Oatmeal with Blueberries

Kidney-Friendly Pancakes (low-sodium, low-phosphorus)

Cinnamon French Toast (with egg whites)

Low-Potassium Smoothie Bowl (with berries and almond milk)

Breakfast Quinoa with Berries and Almonds

Scrambled Tofu with Spinach

Applesauce Pancakes (low-sodium, no butter)

Buckwheat Porridge with Almonds and Berries

Rice Cakes with Peanut Butter and Sliced Apples

Whole Grain English Muffin with Low-Sodium Jam

Cottage Cheese with Strawberries (low-phosphorus option)

Baked Apple with Cinnamon and Oats

Low-Sodium Cornmeal Porridge

Greek Yogurt Parfait (low-sodium, portion-controlled potassium)

Low-Sodium, Low-Potassium Muffins (apple or berry)

Soft-Boiled Egg Whites on Whole Grain Toast

Chia Seed Pudding (made with almond or coconut milk)

Kidney-Safe Berry Smoothie (using almond milk, strawberries, and blueberries)

Low-Sodium Bran Muffins with Cranberries

Egg White and Veggie Scramble

Low Potassium | Mid-Protein | Low Sodium

Servings: 2

Prep Time: 5 minutes

Cook Time: 10 minutes

Ingredients

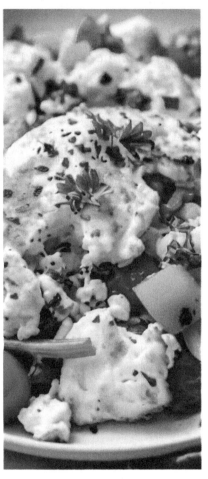

- 4 large egg whites
- 1/4 cup diced bell peppers (low-potassium option)
- 1/4 cup diced onions
- 1/4 cup spinach, chopped
- 1 tsp olive oil
- Salt-free seasoning to taste (optional)
- Fresh parsley, for garnish

Directions

1. Heat the olive oil in a non-stick skillet over medium heat.
2. Add the diced bell peppers and onions to the skillet and sauté for 3-4 minutes until softened.
3. Stir in the chopped spinach and cook for an additional minute until wilted.

4. Pour in the egg whites and gently scramble until fully cooked, about 4-5 minutes.
5. Season with a salt-free seasoning and garnish with fresh parsley.
6. Serve immediately and enjoy!

Nutritional Info Per Serving:

Calories: 80 | Protein: 14g | Carbs: 3g | Sodium: 55mg | Cholesterol: 0mg | Potassium: 150mg | Phosphorus: 20mg

Low-Sodium Oatmeal with Blueberries

Low Sodium | Low Potassium | High Fiber

🍴 Servings: 2

⏱ Prep Time: 5 minutes

🔍 Cook Time: 10 minutes

Ingredients

- 1/2 cup old-fashioned oats
- 1 cup water
- 1/4 cup unsweetened almond milk
- 1/4 cup fresh blueberries
- 1/2 tsp cinnamon
- 1 tsp maple syrup (optional)

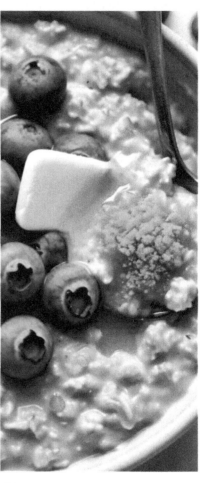

Directions

1. In a small saucepan, bring water to a boil and add the oats.
2. Reduce heat to a simmer and cook the oats for about 5-7 minutes until thickened.
3. Stir in the almond milk and cinnamon, then cook for an additional minute.

4. Remove from heat, top with fresh blueberries, and drizzle with maple syrup if desired.

5. Serve warm and enjoy!

Nutritional Info Per Serving:

Calories: 150 | Protein: 4g | Carbs: 30g | Sodium: 15mg | Cholesterol: 0mg | Potassium: 100mg | Phosphorus: 40mg

Kidney-Friendly Pancakes (Low-Sodium, Low-Phosphorus)

Low Sodium | Low Phosphorus | Low Potassium

⬚ Servings: 2

⏱ Prep Time: 5 minutes

🔍 Cook Time: 10 minutes

Ingredients

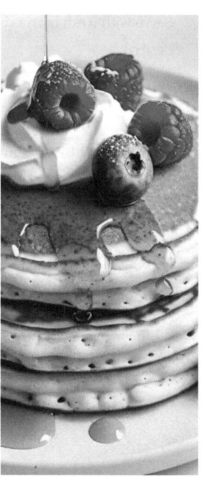

- 1/2 cup all-purpose flour
- 1/4 cup unsweetened almond milk
- 1 egg white
- 1/2 tsp baking powder (low-phosphorus option)
- 1/4 tsp vanilla extract
- 1 tsp olive oil for cooking

Directions

1. In a bowl, whisk together flour, almond milk, egg white, baking powder, and vanilla until smooth.

2. Heat a non-stick skillet over medium heat and lightly coat with olive oil.
3. Pour batter into the skillet, about 1/4 cup per pancake.
4. Cook for 2-3 minutes on each side until golden brown.
5. Serve with fresh berries or a light drizzle of maple syrup if desired.

Nutritional Info Per Serving:

Calories: 140 | Protein: 4g | Carbs: 23g | Sodium: 60mg | Cholesterol: 0mg | Potassium: 50mg | Phosphorus: 40mg

Cinnamon French Toast (with Egg Whites)

Low Sodium | Low Potassium | Low Phosphorus

🗒 Servings: 2

⏱ Prep Time: 5 minutes

🔍 Cook Time: 10 minutes

Ingredients

- 4 slices of whole wheat bread (low sodium)
- 4 large egg whites
- 1/2 tsp cinnamon
- 1/4 cup unsweetened almond milk
- 1 tsp vanilla extract
- 1 tsp olive oil for cooking

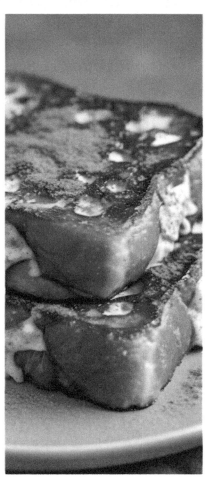

Directions

1. Whisk together egg whites, almond milk, cinnamon, and vanilla in a shallow bowl.
2. Dip each slice of bread into the mixture, making sure both sides are coated.

3. Heat olive oil in a skillet over medium heat and cook each slice for about 2-3 minutes on each side until golden brown.
4. Serve warm with fresh berries or a drizzle of low-sugar syrup.

Nutritional Info Per Serving:

Calories: 160 | Protein: 8g | Carbs: 28g | Sodium: 120mg | Cholesterol: 0mg | Potassium: 100mg | Phosphorus: 70mg

Low-Potassium Smoothie Bowl (with Berries and Almond Milk)

Low Potassium | Low Sodium | Dairy-Free

🍽 Servings: 2

⏲ Prep Time: 5 minutes

🔍 Cook Time: None

Ingredients

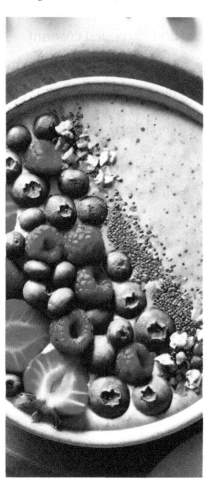

- 1/2 cup unsweetened almond milk
- 1/2 cup frozen mixed berries (blueberries, raspberries)
- 1/4 cup rolled oats
- 1 tbsp chia seeds
- 1 tbsp unsweetened shredded coconut (optional)
- 1 tsp honey or maple syrup (optional)
- Fresh berries for topping

Directions

- In a blender, combine almond milk, frozen mixed berries, oats, and chia seeds.
- Blend until smooth and creamy.
- Pour the smoothie into a bowl and top with fresh berries and shredded coconut.
- Drizzle with honey or maple syrup if desired, and enjoy immediately!

Nutritional Info Per Serving:

Calories: 140 | Protein: 4g | Carbs: 25g | Sodium: 60mg | Cholesterol: 0mg | Potassium: 180mg | Phosphorus: 50mg

Breakfast Quinoa with Berries and Almonds

High Fiber | Low Potassium | Low Sodium

🍽 Servings: 2

⏱ Prep Time: 5 minutes

🔍 Cook Time: 15 minutes

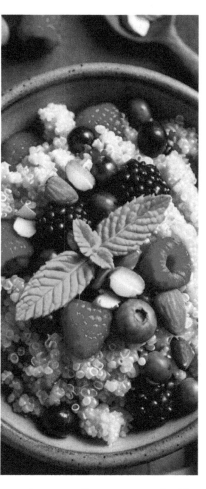

Ingredients

- 1/2 cup quinoa, rinsed
- 1 cup water
- 1/4 cup unsweetened almond milk
- 1/4 cup fresh blueberries
- 1 tbsp sliced almonds
- 1 tsp cinnamon
- 1 tsp honey or maple syrup (optional)

Directions

1. In a small saucepan, bring the quinoa and water to a boil.

2. Reduce the heat to a simmer, cover, and cook for 12-15 minutes, or until the quinoa is tender and water is absorbed.
3. Stir in the almond milk and cinnamon, and cook for another minute.
4. Remove from heat, divide into bowls, and top with fresh blueberries and sliced almonds.
5. Drizzle with honey or maple syrup if desired, and serve warm.

Nutritional Info Per Serving:

Calories: 220 | Protein: 6g | Carbs: 35g | Sodium: 10mg | Cholesterol: 0mg | Potassium: 120mg | Phosphorus: 110mg

Scrambled Tofu with Spinach

Low Potassium | Low Sodium | Vegan

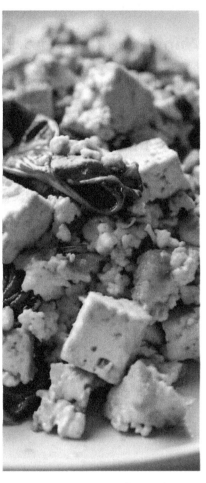

🍽 Servings: 2

⏲ Prep Time: 5 minutes

🔍 Cook Time: 10 minutes

Ingredients

- 1/2 block firm tofu, crumbled
- 1/2 cup fresh spinach, chopped
- 1 tsp olive oil
- 1/4 tsp turmeric
- 1/4 tsp garlic powder
- Salt-free seasoning, to taste
- Fresh parsley, for garnish

Directions

1. Heat the olive oil in a non-stick skillet over medium heat.
2. Add the crumbled tofu and sauté for 3-4 minutes.
3. Stir in the turmeric, garlic powder, and salt-free seasoning, cooking for another minute.

4. Add the chopped spinach and cook until wilted, about 2 minutes.

5. Garnish with fresh parsley and serve warm.

Nutritional Info Per Serving:

Calories: 120 | Protein: 12g | Carbs: 5g | Sodium: 15mg | Cholesterol: 0mg | Potassium: 140mg | Phosphorus: 80mg

Applesauce Pancakes (Low-Sodium, No Butter)

Low Sodium | Low Potassium | Heart-Healthy

🍽 Servings: 2

⏲ Prep Time: 5 minutes

🔍 Cook Time: 10 minutes

Ingredients

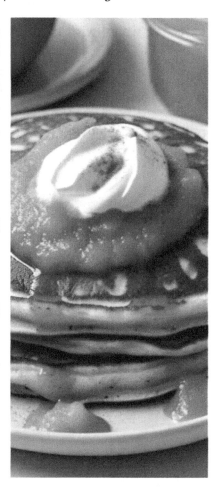

- 1/2 cup whole wheat flour
- 1/4 cup unsweetened applesauce
- 1 egg white
- 1/4 cup unsweetened almond milk
- 1/2 tsp baking powder (low-sodium option)
- 1/4 tsp cinnamon
- 1 tsp olive oil for cooking

Directions

1. In a bowl, whisk together flour, applesauce, egg white, almond milk, baking powder, and cinnamon until smooth.

2. Heat a non-stick skillet over medium heat and lightly coat with olive oil.

3. Pour the batter into the skillet, about 1/4 cup per pancake.

4. Cook for 2-3 minutes on each side until golden brown.

5. Serve warm with fresh fruit or a drizzle of maple syrup if desired.

Nutritional Info Per Serving:

Calories: 160 | Protein: 5g | Carbs: 30g | Sodium: 60mg | Cholesterol: 0mg | Potassium: 90mg | Phosphorus: 40mg

Buckwheat Porridge with Almonds and Berries

Low Sodium | Low Potassium | High Fiber

🍽 Servings: 2

⏱ Prep Time: 5 minutes

🔍 Cook Time: 10 minutes

Ingredients

- 1/2 cup buckwheat groats
- 1 cup water
- 1/4 cup unsweetened almond milk
- 1/4 cup fresh raspberries
- 1 tbsp sliced almonds
- 1 tsp honey or maple syrup (optional)

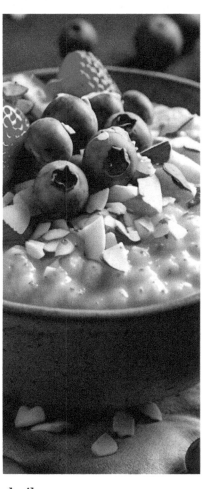

Directions

1. In a small saucepan, bring the buckwheat and water to a boil.
2. Reduce the heat and simmer for 10 minutes, stirring occasionally, until the buckwheat is tender.

3. Stir in the almond milk and cook for another minute.
4. Remove from heat and top with fresh raspberries and sliced almonds.
5. Drizzle with honey or maple syrup if desired, and serve warm.

Nutritional Info Per Serving:

Calories: 180 | Protein: 5g | Carbs: 32g | Sodium: 15mg | Cholesterol: 0mg | Potassium: 120mg | Phosphorus: 80mg

Rice Cakes with Peanut Butter and Sliced Apples

Low Sodium | Low Potassium | Heart-Healthy

🍽 Servings: 2

⏱ Prep Time: 5 minutes

🔍 Cook Time: None

Ingredients

- 4 unsalted rice cakes
- 2 tbsp peanut butter (unsalted, natural)
- 1 small apple, thinly sliced
- 1/2 tsp cinnamon (optional)

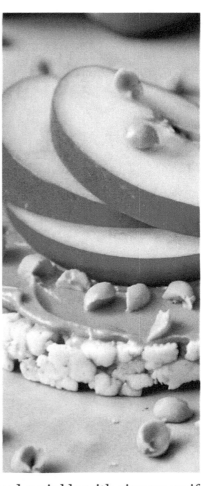

Directions

1. Spread 1 tbsp of peanut butter evenly on two rice cakes.
2. Top each with sliced apples and sprinkle with cinnamon if desired.
3. Serve immediately and enjoy!

Nutritional Info Per Serving:

Calories: 180 | Protein: 6g | Carbs: 26g | Sodium: 40mg | Cholesterol: 0mg | Potassium: 150mg | Phosphorus: 80mg

Whole Grain English Muffin with Low-Sodium Jam

Low Sodium | Low Potassium | High Fiber

🍽 Servings: 2

⏱ Prep Time: 2 minutes

🔍 Cook Time: 5 minutes

Ingredients

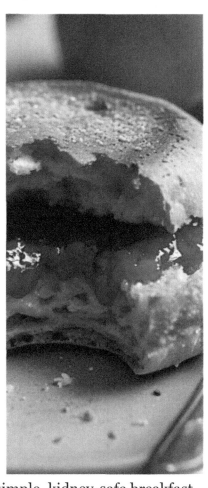

- 2 whole grain English muffins (low sodium)
- 2 tbsp low-sodium jam (such as strawberry or apricot)

Directions

1. Split and toast the whole grain English muffins.
2. Spread 1 tbsp of low-sodium jam on each half.
3. Serve warm and enjoy as a simple, kidney-safe breakfast.

Nutritional Info Per Serving:

Calories: 160 | Protein: 4g | Carbs: 32g | Sodium: 60mg | Cholesterol: 0mg | Potassium: 80mg | Phosphorus: 50mg

Cottage Cheese with Strawberries (Low-Phosphorus Option)

Low Sodium | Low Phosphorus | Low Potassium

Servings: 2

Prep Time: 5 minutes

Cook Time: None

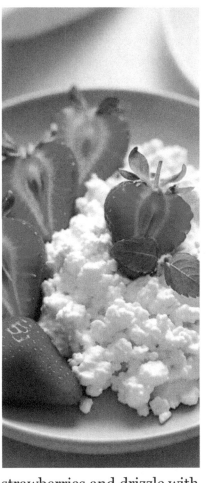

Ingredients

- 1/2 cup low-phosphorus cottage cheese (kidney-friendly brand)
- 1/4 cup fresh strawberries, sliced
- 1 tsp honey or maple syrup (optional)

Directions

1. Divide the cottage cheese between two bowls.
2. Top each serving with sliced strawberries and drizzle with honey if desired.
3. Serve immediately for a quick and refreshing breakfast.

Nutritional Info Per Serving:

Calories: 90 | Protein: 6g | Carbs: 8g | Sodium: 80mg |
Cholesterol: 5mg | Potassium: 140mg | Phosphorus: 70mg

Baked Apple with Cinnamon and Oats

Low Sodium | Low Potassium | High Fiber

🍽 Servings: 2

⏱ Prep Time: 5 minutes

🔍 Cook Time: 20 minutes

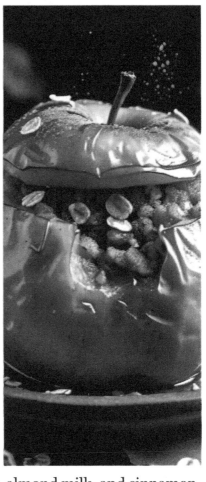

Ingredients

- 2 small apples, cored
- 1/4 cup rolled oats
- 1/2 tsp cinnamon
- 1 tbsp unsweetened almond milk
- 1 tsp honey or maple syrup (optional)

Directions

1. Preheat the oven to 350°F (175°C).
2. In a small bowl, mix the oats, almond milk, and cinnamon.
3. Stuff each apple with the oat mixture and place them in a baking dish.
4. Bake for 20 minutes until the apples are tender.

5. Drizzle with honey or maple syrup if desired, and serve warm.

Nutritional Info Per Serving:

Calories: 120 | Protein: 2g | Carbs: 28g | Sodium: 5mg | Cholesterol: 0mg | Potassium: 150mg | Phosphorus: 30mg

Low-Sodium Cornmeal Porridge

Low Sodium | Low Phosphorus | Low Potassium

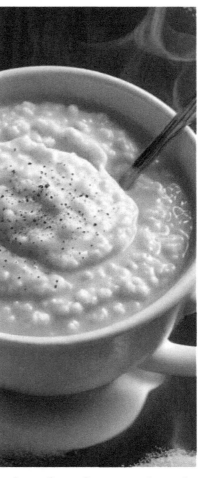

🍽 Servings: 2

⏱ Prep Time: 5 minutes

🔍 Cook Time: 10 minutes

Ingredients

- 1/2 cup cornmeal
- 1 1/2 cups water
- 1/4 cup unsweetened almond milk
- 1 tsp cinnamon
- 1 tsp honey or maple syrup (optional)

Directions

1. In a small saucepan, bring water to a boil.
2. Slowly whisk in the cornmeal, reduce heat, and cook, stirring frequently, for 8-10 minutes until thickened.
3. Stir in the almond milk and cinnamon, and cook for another minute.

4. Serve warm with a drizzle of honey or maple syrup if desired.

Nutritional Info Per Serving:

Calories: 150 | Protein: 2g | Carbs: 32g | Sodium: 5mg | Cholesterol: 0mg | Potassium: 70mg | Phosphorus: 20mg

Greek Yogurt Parfait (Low-Sodium, Portion-Controlled Potassium)

Low Sodium | Mid-Protein | Heart-Healthy

🍶 Servings: 2

⏱ Prep Time: 5 minutes

🔍 Cook Time: None

Ingredients

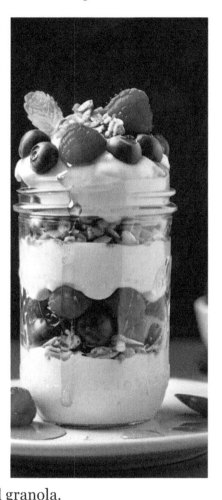

- 1/2 cup plain Greek yogurt (low-sodium)
- 1/4 cup fresh blueberries
- 2 tbsp granola (low-sodium, low-potassium)
- 1 tsp honey or maple syrup (optional)

Directions

1. In two serving glasses or bowls, layer the Greek yogurt with blueberries and granola.
2. Drizzle with honey or maple syrup if desired.

3. Serve immediately and enjoy this simple, protein-rich breakfast.

Nutritional Info Per Serving:

Calories: 120 | Protein: 8g | Carbs: 18g | Sodium: 50mg | Cholesterol: 5mg | Potassium: 150mg | Phosphorus: 100mg

Low-Sodium, Low-Potassium Muffins (Apple or Berry)

Low Sodium | Low Potassium | Heart-Healthy

🍴 Servings: 2

⏱ Prep Time: 10 minutes

🔍 Cook Time: 15 minutes

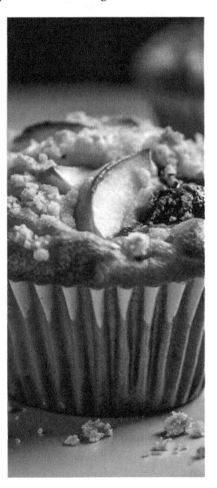

Ingredients

- 1/2 cup all-purpose flour
- 1/4 cup unsweetened applesauce (or fresh berries)
- 1/4 cup unsweetened almond milk
- 1 egg white
- 1/2 tsp baking powder (low-sodium)
- 1/4 tsp vanilla extract
- 1 tsp olive oil

Directions

1. Preheat the oven to 350°F (175°C) and grease a muffin tin.

2. In a bowl, whisk together the flour, applesauce or berries, almond milk, egg white, baking powder, and vanilla extract.
3. Pour the batter into the muffin tin and bake for 12-15 minutes, or until a toothpick comes out clean.
4. Allow to cool before serving.

Nutritional Info Per Serving:

Calories: 150 | Protein: 3g | Carbs: 28g | Sodium: 50mg | Cholesterol: 0mg | Potassium: 60mg | Phosphorus: 40mg

Soft-Boiled Egg Whites on Whole Grain Toast

Low Potassium | Low Sodium | Mid-Protein

🍽 Servings: 2

⏱ Prep Time: 5 minutes

🔍 Cook Time: 6 minutes

Ingredients

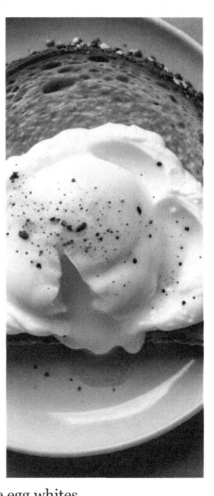

- 4 large egg whites
- 2 slices whole grain bread (low sodium)
- 1 tsp olive oil or butter (optional)
- Fresh parsley or chives for garnish

Directions

1. Bring a small pot of water to a boil. Lower the heat to a simmer and gently add the egg whites.
2. Cook for 6 minutes for soft-boiled egg whites.

3. Toast the whole grain bread and lightly spread with olive oil or butter if desired.

4. Place the soft-boiled egg whites on top of the toast and garnish with fresh parsley or chives.

5. Serve warm and enjoy.

Nutritional Info Per Serving:

Calories: 150 | Protein: 12g | Carbs: 18g | Sodium: 80mg | Cholesterol: 0mg | Potassium: 130mg | Phosphorus: 40mg

Chia Seed Pudding (made with almond or coconut milk)

Low Potassium | Low Sodium | High Fiber

🍴 Servings: 2

⏱ Prep Time: 5 minutes

🔍 Cook Time: 4 hours (chill time)

Ingredients

- 1/4 cup chia seeds
- 1 cup unsweetened almond milk (or coconut milk)
- 1 tsp vanilla extract
- 1 tsp honey or maple syrup (optional)
- Fresh berries for topping (optional)

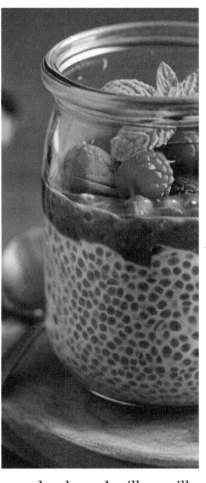

Directions

1. In a bowl, whisk together chia seeds, almond milk, vanilla extract, and honey or maple syrup (if using).

2. Stir well and cover the bowl. Refrigerate for at least 4 hours, or overnight, until the mixture thickens into a pudding-like consistency.

3. Serve chilled with fresh berries on top if desired.

Nutritional Info Per Serving:

Calories: 140 | Protein: 4g | Carbs: 12g | Sodium: 50mg | Cholesterol: 0mg | Potassium: 140mg | Phosphorus: 90mg

Kidney-Safe Berry Smoothie (using almond milk, strawberries, and blueberries)

Low Potassium | Low Sodium | Dairy-Free

🍴 Servings: 2

⏱ Prep Time: 5 minutes

🔍 Cook Time: None

Ingredients

- 1/2 cup unsweetened almond milk
- 1/4 cup fresh or frozen strawberries
- 1/4 cup fresh or frozen blueberries
- 1 tbsp chia seeds (optional)
- 1 tsp honey or maple syrup (optional)

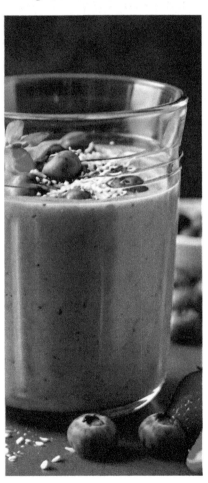

Directions

1. In a blender, combine almond milk, strawberries, blueberries, and chia seeds (if using).

2. Blend until smooth and creamy.

3. Pour into glasses and drizzle with honey or maple syrup if desired.

4. Serve immediately.

Nutritional Info Per Serving:

Calories: 100 | Protein: 2g | Carbs: 18g | Sodium: 30mg | Cholesterol: 0mg | Potassium: 120mg | Phosphorus: 40mg

Low-Sodium Bran Muffins with Cranberries

Low Sodium | High Fiber | Low Potassium

🍴 Servings: 2

⏱ Prep Time: 10 minutes

🔍 Cook Time: 15 minutes

Ingredients

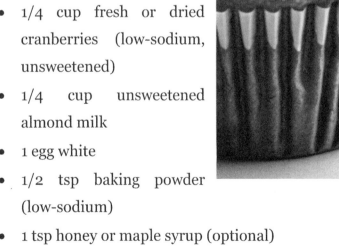

- 1/2 cup wheat bran
- 1/2 cup whole wheat flour
- 1/4 cup unsweetened applesauce
- 1/4 cup fresh or dried cranberries (low-sodium, unsweetened)
- 1/4 cup unsweetened almond milk
- 1 egg white
- 1/2 tsp baking powder (low-sodium)
- 1 tsp honey or maple syrup (optional)

Directions

1. Preheat the oven to 350°F (175°C) and grease a muffin tin.
2. In a bowl, mix wheat bran, flour, baking powder, applesauce, cranberries, almond milk, and egg white until smooth.
3. Pour the batter into the muffin tin and bake for 12-15 minutes, or until a toothpick comes out clean.
4. Allow to cool before serving.

Nutritional Info Per Serving:

Calories: 160 | Protein: 4g | Carbs: 28g | Sodium: 50mg | Cholesterol: 0mg | Potassium: 100mg | Phosphorus: 60mg

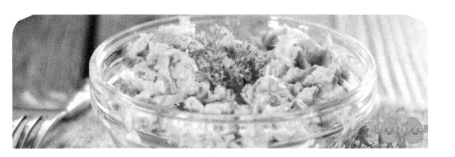

CHAPTER 6: LUNCH RECIPES FOR STAGE 3 CKD

Grilled Chicken and Veggie Wrap (low-sodium tortilla, kidney-safe veggies)

Tuna Salad (low-sodium tuna, light mayo, with whole wheat bread)

Quinoa Salad with Cucumbers and Olive Oil Dressing

Grilled Chicken Caesar Salad (with low-sodium dressing)

Kidney-Friendly Turkey Sandwich (low-sodium turkey, whole wheat bread)

Lentil Soup (low-sodium broth, kidney-friendly veggies)

Grilled Veggie Sandwich with Hummus

Low-Sodium Chicken Soup with Rice

Couscous Salad with Parsley and Lemon

Low-Potassium Pasta Salad (using white pasta, olive oil, kidney-safe veggies)

Egg Salad (with egg whites, low-sodium mayo, on whole wheat toast)

Baked Tilapia with Brown Rice and Steamed Veggies

Chicken Salad with Apples and Low-Fat Dressing

Vegetable Stir-Fry (kidney-friendly veggies, low-sodium soy sauce alternative)

Low-Sodium Veggie Soup (with kidney-safe **Ingredients** like carrots, celery)

Open-Faced Turkey Sandwich (whole wheat bread, low-sodium turkey)

Low-Sodium Macaroni Salad (with olive oil dressing)

Baked Salmon with Lemon and Steamed Veggies

Couscous Bowl with Grilled Chicken and Zucchini

Bean and Veggie Salad (kidney-safe beans like green beans, low-sodium dressing)

Grilled Chicken and Veggie Wrap (Low-Sodium Tortilla, Kidney-Safe Veggies)

Low Sodium | Low Potassium | Mid-Protein

🍴 Servings: 2

⏱ Prep Time: 10 minutes

🔍 Cook Time: 10 minutes

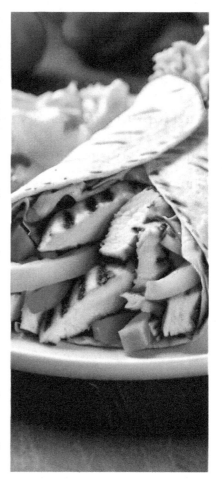

Ingredients

- 2 low-sodium whole wheat tortillas
- 1 small chicken breast, grilled and sliced
- 1/4 cup diced bell peppers
- 1/4 cup shredded lettuce
- 1/4 cup cucumber slices
- 1 tbsp hummus (optional, low-sodium)
- Fresh parsley or cilantro for garnish

Directions

1. Grill the chicken breast and slice it into thin strips.

2. Warm the tortillas in a dry pan over medium heat for about 1 minute on each side.
3. Spread a thin layer of hummus on each tortilla.
4. Add the grilled chicken, bell peppers, shredded lettuce, and cucumber slices.
5. Roll up the wraps, garnish with fresh parsley or cilantro, and serve immediately.

Nutritional Info Per Serving:

Calories: 230 | Protein: 22g | Carbs: 22g | Sodium: 150mg | Cholesterol: 50mg | Potassium: 220mg | Phosphorus: 180mg

Tuna Salad (Low-Sodium Tuna, Light Mayo, with Whole Wheat Bread)

Low Sodium | Mid-Protein | Heart-Healthy

🍽 Servings: 2

⏱ Prep Time: 10 minutes

🔍 Cook Time: None

Ingredients

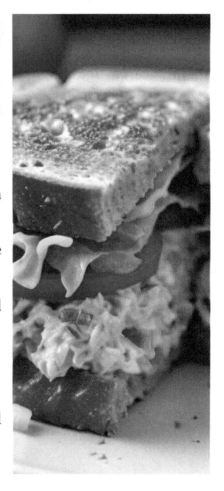

- 1 can (5 oz) low-sodium tuna, drained
- 2 tbsp light mayonnaise (low-sodium)
- 1 tsp Dijon mustard (optional)
- 1/4 cup diced celery
- 1/4 cup diced cucumber
- 4 slices whole wheat bread (low sodium)

Directions

1. In a mixing bowl, combine the drained tuna, mayonnaise, Dijon mustard (if using), diced celery, and cucumber.

2. Stir well to combine.

3. Spread the tuna mixture evenly over two slices of bread, then top with the remaining slices.

4. Serve immediately, or refrigerate for later.

Nutritional Info Per Serving:

Calories: 200 | Protein: 22g | Carbs: 24g | Sodium: 180mg | Cholesterol: 30mg | Potassium: 150mg | Phosphorus: 220mg

Quinoa Salad with Cucumbers and Olive Oil Dressing

Low Sodium | Low Potassium | High Fiber

🍴 Servings: 2

⏱ Prep Time: 10 minutes

🔍 Cook Time: 15 minutes

Ingredients

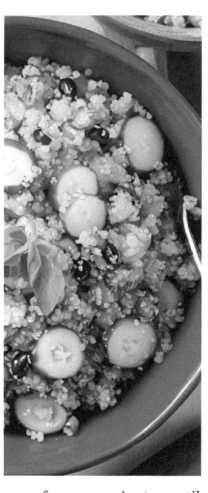

- 1/2 cup quinoa, rinsed
- 1 cup water
- 1/4 cup diced cucumber
- 1/4 cup diced bell peppers
- 1 tbsp olive oil
- 1 tsp lemon juice
- Fresh parsley for garnish

Directions

1. In a saucepan, bring water to a boil and add the quinoa. Reduce heat and simmer for 12-15 minutes until the quinoa is tender and water is absorbed.

2. Allow the quinoa to cool slightly, then mix in the diced cucumber, bell peppers, olive oil, and lemon juice.

3. Garnish with fresh parsley and serve chilled or at room temperature.

Nutritional Info Per Serving:

Calories: 210 | Protein: 6g | Carbs: 30g | Sodium: 10mg | Cholesterol: 0mg | Potassium: 160mg | Phosphorus: 130mg

Grilled Chicken Caesar Salad (with Low-Sodium Dressing)

Low Sodium | Mid-Protein | Low Potassium

🍴 Servings: 2

⏱ Prep Time: 10 minutes

🔍 Cook Time: 10 minutes

Ingredients

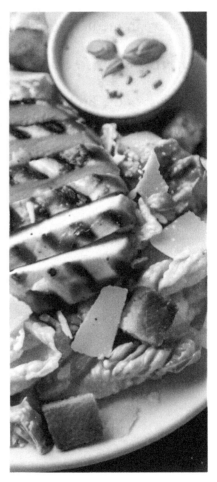

- 1 small chicken breast, grilled and sliced
- 2 cups romaine lettuce, chopped
- 1/4 cup low-sodium Caesar dressing
- 1 tbsp Parmesan cheese (optional)
- 1/4 cup croutons (low-sodium option)

Directions

1. Grill the chicken breast and slice it thinly.

2. In a large bowl, toss the chopped romaine lettuce with the low-sodium Caesar dressing.
3. Top the salad with grilled chicken, Parmesan cheese (if using), and croutons.
4. Serve immediately and enjoy!

Nutritional Info Per Serving:

Calories: 250 | Protein: 22g | Carbs: 10g | Sodium: 180mg | Cholesterol: 45mg | Potassium: 200mg | Phosphorus: 180mg

Kidney-Friendly Turkey Sandwich (Low-Sodium Turkey, Whole Wheat Bread)

Low Sodium | Low Potassium | High Fiber

🔲 Servings: 2

⏱ Prep Time: 5 minutes

🔍 Cook Time: None

Ingredients

- 4 slices low-sodium turkey breast
- 4 slices whole wheat bread (low sodium)
- 2 tbsp low-sodium mustard
- 1/4 cup shredded lettuce
- 1/4 cup sliced cucumber

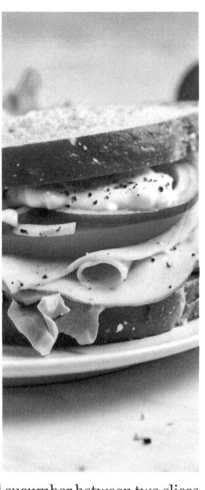

Directions

1. Spread mustard on each slice of bread.
2. Layer the turkey, lettuce, and cucumber between two slices of bread.
3. Serve immediately or pack for lunch.

Nutritional Info Per Serving:

Calories: 180 | Protein: 18g | Carbs: 24g | Sodium: 160mg | Cholesterol: 25mg | Potassium: 150mg | Phosphorus: 150mg

Lentil Soup (Low-Sodium Broth, Kidney-Friendly Veggies)

Low Sodium | High Fiber | Heart-Healthy

🍴 Servings: 2

⏱ Prep Time: 10 minutes

🔍 Cook Time: 25 minutes

Ingredients

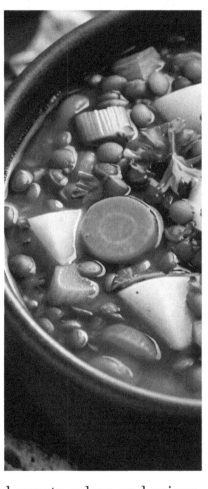

- 1/2 cup dried lentils, rinsed
- 3 cups low-sodium vegetable broth
- 1/4 cup diced carrots
- 1/4 cup diced celery
- 1/4 cup diced onions
- 1 tsp olive oil
- Fresh parsley for garnish

Directions

1. In a large pot, heat olive oil over medium heat. Add diced carrots, celery, and onions, and sauté for 5 minutes.
2. Add the lentils and vegetable broth, and bring to a boil.

3. Reduce the heat, cover, and simmer for 20 minutes, or until lentils are tender.
4. Garnish with fresh parsley and serve hot.

Nutritional Info Per Serving:

Calories: 220 | Protein: 12g | Carbs: 38g | Sodium: 90mg | Cholesterol: 0mg | Potassium: 320mg | Phosphorus: 180mg

Grilled Veggie Sandwich with Hummus

Low Sodium | Low Potassium | High Fiber

Servings: 2

Prep Time: 10 minutes

Cook Time: 10 minutes

Ingredients

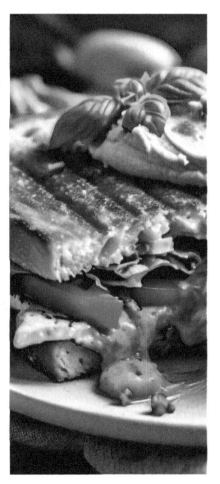

- 4 slices whole wheat bread (low sodium)
- 1/4 cup hummus (low sodium)
- 1/2 cup grilled zucchini, thinly sliced
- 1/2 cup grilled bell peppers, thinly sliced
- 1 tbsp olive oil for grilling
- Fresh parsley or cilantro for garnish

Directions

1. Brush zucchini and bell peppers with olive oil and grill for 5 minutes on each side until soft and slightly charred.
2. Spread hummus on each slice of bread.

3. Layer the grilled veggies between the bread slices and garnish with parsley or cilantro.

4. Serve warm or cold.

Nutritional Info Per Serving:

Calories: 250 | Protein: 8g | Carbs: 36g | Sodium: 150mg | Cholesterol: 0mg | Potassium: 250mg | Phosphorus: 120mg

Low-Sodium Chicken Soup with Rice

Low Sodium | Mid-Protein | Heart-Healthy

🍽 Servings: 2

⏱ Prep Time: 10 minutes

🔍 Cook Time: 25 minutes

Ingredients

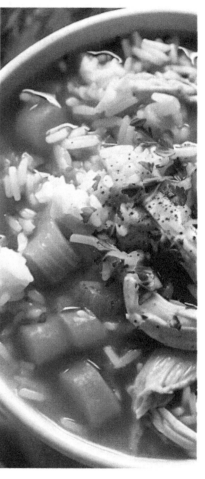

- 1 small chicken breast, diced
- 3 cups low-sodium chicken broth
- 1/4 cup brown rice, rinsed
- 1/4 cup diced carrots
- 1/4 cup diced celery
- 1 tsp olive oil
- Fresh parsley for garnish

Directions

1. Heat olive oil in a large pot over medium heat. Add diced chicken and sauté for 5 minutes until browned.
2. Add diced carrots and celery and cook for an additional 5 minutes.

3. Stir in chicken broth and brown rice. Bring to a boil, then reduce heat and simmer for 20 minutes until rice is tender.

4. Garnish with fresh parsley and serve warm.

Nutritional Info Per Serving:

Calories: 230 | Protein: 22g | Carbs: 28g | Sodium: 120mg | Cholesterol: 45mg | Potassium: 220mg | Phosphorus: 180mg

Couscous Salad with Parsley and Lemon

Low Sodium | Low Potassium | High Fiber

🍱 Servings: 2

⏱ Prep Time: 10 minutes

🔍 Cook Time: 5 minutes

Ingredients

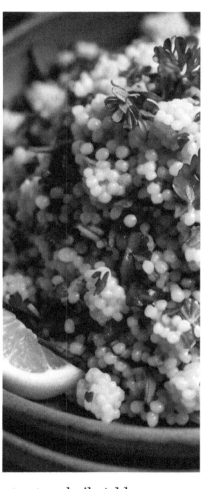

- 1/2 cup couscous
- 1 cup water
- 1/4 cup diced cucumber
- 1/4 cup diced tomatoes (optional, low-potassium variety)
- 1 tbsp olive oil
- 1 tbsp lemon juice
- Fresh parsley for garnish

Directions

1. In a small saucepan, bring water to a boil. Add couscous, cover, and remove from heat. Let sit for 5 minutes.

2. Fluff couscous with a fork, then mix in diced cucumber, tomatoes (if using), olive oil, and lemon juice.
3. Garnish with fresh parsley and serve chilled or at room temperature.

Nutritional Info Per Serving:

Calories: 190 | Protein: 5g | Carbs: 32g | Sodium: 10mg | Cholesterol: 0mg | Potassium: 150mg | Phosphorus: 80mg

Low-Potassium Pasta Salad (using white pasta, olive oil, kidney-safe veggies)

Low Potassium | Low Sodium | Heart-Healthy

🍽 Servings: 2

⏱ Prep Time: 10 minutes

🔍 Cook Time: 10 minutes

Ingredients

- 1/2 cup white pasta (low-sodium variety)
- 1/4 cup diced cucumber
- 1/4 cup diced bell peppers
- 1 tbsp olive oil
- 1 tsp lemon juice
- Fresh basil for garnish

Directions

1. Cook the pasta according to package instructions, then drain and rinse under cold water.

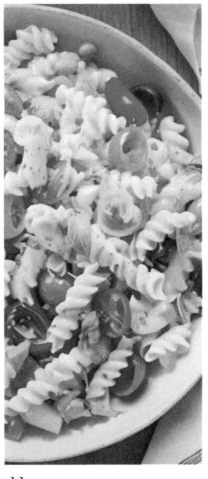

2. In a large bowl, mix the cooked pasta with diced cucumber, bell peppers, olive oil, and lemon juice.

3. Garnish with fresh basil and serve cold.

Nutritional Info Per Serving:

Calories: 220 | Protein: 6g | Carbs: 34g | Sodium: 15mg | Cholesterol: 0mg | Potassium: 140mg | Phosphorus: 80mg

Egg Salad (with Egg Whites, Low-Sodium Mayo, on Whole Wheat Toast)

Low Sodium | Low Potassium | Mid-Protein

🍽 Servings: 2

⏱ Prep Time: 5 minutes

🔍 Cook Time: 10 minutes

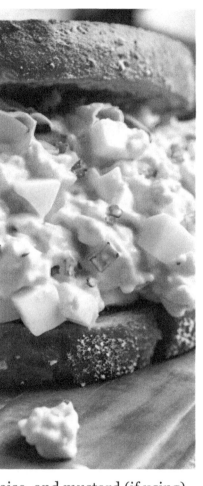

Ingredients

- 4 large egg whites, boiled and chopped
- 2 tbsp low-sodium mayonnaise
- 1/4 tsp mustard (optional)
- 4 slices whole wheat toast (low sodium)
- Fresh parsley for garnish

Directions

1. In a bowl, combine chopped egg whites, mayonnaise, and mustard (if using).
2. Spread the egg salad on whole wheat toast.
3. Garnish with fresh parsley and serve immediately.

Nutritional Info Per Serving:

Calories: 200 | Protein: 10g | Carbs: 24g | Sodium: 160mg | Cholesterol: 0mg | Potassium: 130mg | Phosphorus: 120mg

Baked Tilapia with Brown Rice and Steamed Veggies

Low Sodium | Low Potassium | High Protein

🍴 Servings: 2

⏱ Prep Time: 10 minutes

🔍 Cook Time: 20 minutes

Ingredients

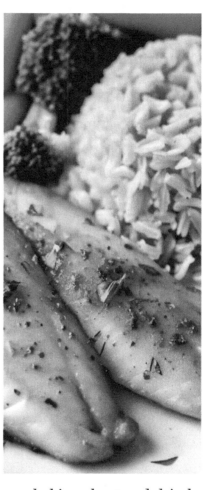

- 2 small tilapia fillets
- 1/2 cup brown rice, rinsed
- 1 cup low-sodium vegetable broth
- 1/4 cup diced zucchini
- 1/4 cup diced carrots
- 1 tsp olive oil
- Fresh parsley for garnish

Directions

1. Preheat the oven to 375°F (190°C). Place tilapia fillets on a baking sheet and drizzle with olive oil.
2. Bake for 15-20 minutes until the fish is cooked through.

3. In a saucepan, bring vegetable broth to a boil, add the brown rice, cover, and simmer for 15 minutes.
4. Steam zucchini and carrots until tender.
5. Serve the baked tilapia with brown rice and steamed veggies, garnished with fresh parsley.

Nutritional Info Per Serving:

Calories: 300 | Protein: 26g | Carbs: 32g | Sodium: 120mg | Cholesterol: 55mg | Potassium: 250mg | Phosphorus: 230mg

Chicken Salad with Apples and Low-Fat Dressing

Low Sodium | Low Potassium | Heart-Healthy

🍽 Servings: 2

⏱ Prep Time: 10 minutes

🔍 Cook Time: None

Ingredients

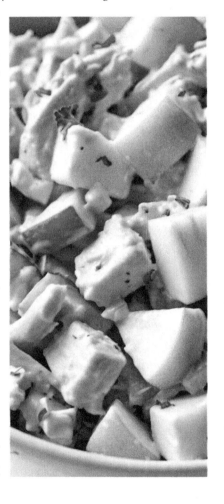

- 1 small chicken breast, grilled and diced
- 1/2 cup diced apples
- 1/4 cup low-fat Greek yogurt (unsweetened)
- 1 tsp lemon juice
- Fresh parsley for garnish

Directions

1. In a bowl, mix diced chicken, apples, Greek yogurt, and lemon juice.
2. Toss well to combine and garnish with fresh parsley.
3. Serve chilled or at room temperature.

Nutritional Info Per Serving:

Calories: 180 | Protein: 20g | Carbs: 16g | Sodium: 80mg | Cholesterol: 45mg | Potassium: 160mg | Phosphorus: 180mg

Vegetable Stir-Fry (Kidney-Friendly Veggies, Low-Sodium Soy Sauce Alternative)

Low Sodium | Low Potassium | Vegan

🍽 Servings: 2

⏱ Prep Time: 10 minutes

🔍 Cook Time: 10 minutes

Ingredients

- 1/2 cup sliced zucchini
- 1/2 cup sliced bell peppers
- 1/4 cup sliced carrots
- 1/4 cup sliced onions
- 1 tsp olive oil
- 1 tbsp low-sodium soy sauce alternative (or tamari)
- 1 tsp sesame seeds (optional)

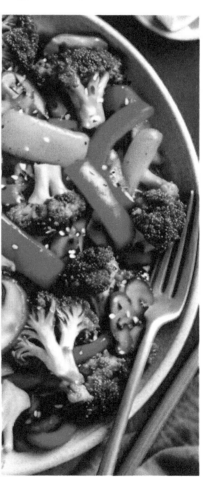

Directions

1. Heat olive oil in a non-stick skillet over medium heat.

2. Add zucchini, bell peppers, carrots, and onions to the skillet. Stir-fry for 5-7 minutes until the veggies are tender.

3. Add the low-sodium soy sauce alternative and stir to coat the vegetables evenly.

4. Sprinkle with sesame seeds, if desired, and serve immediately.

Nutritional Info Per Serving:

Calories: 140 | Protein: 3g | Carbs: 18g | Sodium: 80mg | Cholesterol: 0mg | Potassium: 250mg | Phosphorus: 50mg

Low-Sodium Veggie Soup (with Kidney-Safe Ingredients like Carrots, Celery)

Low Sodium | Low Potassium | High Fiber

🍽 Servings: 2

⏱ Prep Time: 10 minutes

🔍 Cook Time: 20 minutes

Ingredients

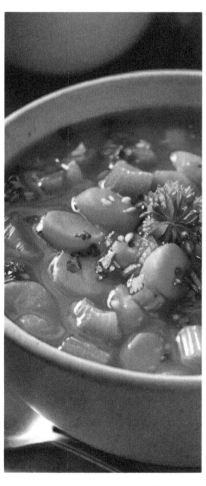

- 1/4 cup diced carrots
- 1/4 cup diced celery
- 1/4 cup diced onions
- 1/2 cup low-sodium vegetable broth
- 1/4 cup chopped zucchini
- 1 tsp olive oil
- Fresh parsley for garnish

Directions

1. Heat olive oil in a pot over medium heat. Add carrots, celery, and onions, and sauté for 5 minutes.

2. Add the low-sodium vegetable broth and chopped zucchini. Bring to a boil, then reduce heat and simmer for 15 minutes.

3. Garnish with fresh parsley and serve hot.

Nutritional Info Per Serving:

Calories: 120 | Protein: 2g | Carbs: 20g | Sodium: 60mg | Cholesterol: 0mg | Potassium: 140mg | Phosphorus: 40mg

Open-Faced Turkey Sandwich (Whole Wheat Bread, Low-Sodium Turkey)

Low Sodium | Mid-Protein | High Fiber

Servings: 2

Prep Time: 5 minutes

Cook Time: None

Ingredients

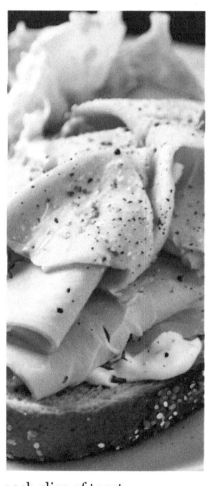

- 4 slices low-sodium turkey breast
- 2 slices whole wheat bread (low sodium)
- 1/4 cup shredded lettuce
- 1 tbsp light mayonnaise (low sodium)

Directions

1. Toast the whole wheat bread slices.
2. Spread light mayonnaise on each slice of toast.
3. Layer with low-sodium turkey breast and shredded lettuce.

4. Serve open-faced and enjoy.

Nutritional Info Per Serving:

Calories: 180 | Protein: 16g | Carbs: 22g | Sodium: 120mg | Cholesterol: 25mg | Potassium: 150mg | Phosphorus: 140mg

Low-Sodium Macaroni Salad (with Olive Oil Dressing)

Low Sodium | Low Potassium | High Fiber

[🍽] Servings: 2

[⏱] Prep Time: 10 minutes

[🔍] Cook Time: 10 minutes

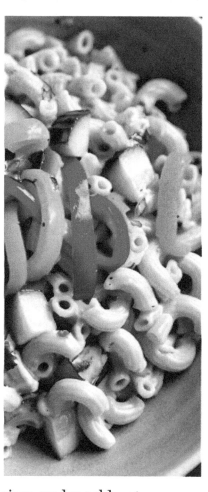

Ingredients

- 1/2 cup elbow macaroni (low sodium)
- 1/4 cup diced cucumber
- 1/4 cup diced bell peppers
- 1 tbsp olive oil
- 1 tsp lemon juice
- Fresh parsley for garnish

Directions

1. Cook the macaroni according to package instructions, then drain and rinse under cold water.
2. In a large bowl, mix the cooked macaroni with diced cucumber, bell peppers, olive oil, and lemon juice.

3. Garnish with fresh parsley and serve chilled.

Nutritional Info Per Serving:

Calories: 200 | Protein: 5g | Carbs: 34g | Sodium: 40mg |
Cholesterol: 0mg | Potassium: 120mg | Phosphorus: 60mg

Baked Salmon with Lemon and Steamed Veggies

Low Sodium | Low Potassium | High Protein

[icon] Servings: 2

[icon] Prep Time: 10 minutes

[icon] Cook Time: 15 minutes

Ingredients

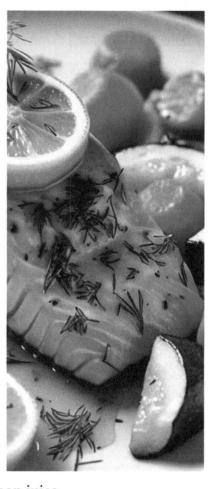

- 2 small salmon fillets
- 1/4 cup steamed zucchini
- 1/4 cup steamed carrots
- 1 tsp olive oil
- 1 tbsp lemon juice
- Fresh parsley for garnish

Directions

1. Preheat the oven to 375°F (190°C). Place the salmon fillets on a baking sheet and drizzle with olive oil and lemon juice.
2. Bake for 12-15 minutes until the salmon is cooked through.
3. Steam the zucchini and carrots until tender.

4. Serve the baked salmon with steamed veggies, garnished with fresh parsley.

Nutritional Info Per Serving:

Calories: 280 | Protein: 24g | Carbs: 12g | Sodium: 90mg | Cholesterol: 60mg | Potassium: 280mg | Phosphorus: 220mg

Couscous Bowl with Grilled Chicken and Zucchini

Low Sodium | Low Potassium | High Protein

🍽 Servings: 2

⏱ Prep Time: 10 minutes

🔍 Cook Time: 20 minutes

Ingredients

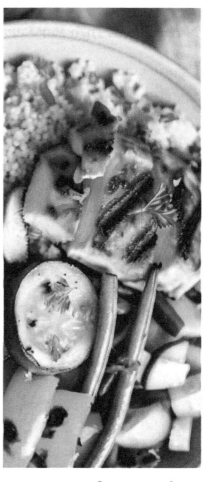

- 1/2 cup couscous
- 1 small chicken breast, grilled and sliced
- 1/4 cup grilled zucchini, sliced
- 1 tbsp olive oil
- 1 tsp lemon juice
- Fresh parsley for garnish

Directions

1. In a small saucepan, bring water to a boil. Add couscous, cover, and remove from heat. Let sit for 5 minutes.
2. Grill the chicken breast and slice thinly.

3. In a large bowl, mix the cooked couscous with grilled zucchini, olive oil, and lemon juice.

4. Top with grilled chicken and garnish with fresh parsley. Serve warm or chilled.

Nutritional Info Per Serving:

Calories: 260 | Protein: 22g | Carbs: 28g | Sodium: 80mg | Cholesterol: 45mg | Potassium: 200mg | Phosphorus: 180mg

Bean and Veggie Salad (Kidney-Safe Beans like Green Beans, Low-Sodium Dressing)

Low Sodium | Low Potassium | High Fiber

Servings: 2

Prep Time: 10 minutes

Cook Time: None

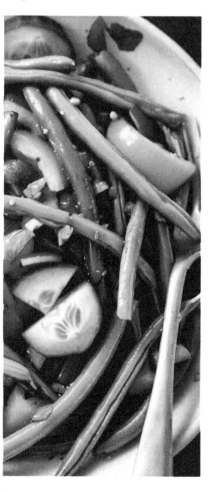

Ingredients

- 1/2 cup green beans (steamed and cooled)
- 1/4 cup diced bell peppers
- 1/4 cup diced cucumbers
- 1 tbsp olive oil
- 1 tsp lemon juice
- Fresh parsley for garnish

Directions

1. In a large bowl, mix the steamed green beans, diced bell peppers, and cucumbers.
2. Drizzle with olive oil and lemon juice.

3. Garnish with fresh parsley and serve chilled.

Nutritional Info Per Serving:

Calories: 150 | Protein: 4g | Carbs: 16g | Sodium: 50mg | Cholesterol: 0mg | Potassium: 180mg | Phosphorus: 70mg

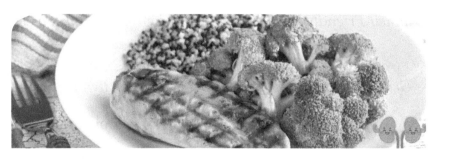

CHAPTER 7: DINNER RECIPES FOR STAGE 3 CKD

Herb-Roasted Chicken with Quinoa

Grilled Salmon with Steamed Asparagus

Baked Chicken Thighs with Roasted Carrots

Turkey Meatballs with Kidney-Safe Tomato Sauce

Pork Tenderloin with Steamed Broccoli

Grilled Tilapia with Lemon and Quinoa

Low-Sodium Chicken Stir-Fry with Brown Rice

Kidney-Friendly Shepherd's Pie (using lean ground beef, no-salt mashed cauliflower)

Baked Cod with Roasted Zucchini and Brown Rice

Kidney-Friendly Veggie Pizza (using low-potassium sauce, kidney-safe veggies)

Grilled Chicken with Couscous and Roasted Red Peppers

Stuffed Bell Peppers (with lean turkey, brown rice)

Grilled Turkey Burgers (low-sodium, served with a side of mixed greens)

Baked Lemon Herb Chicken with Steamed Carrots

Chicken and Rice Casserole (low-sodium version with kidney-friendly vegetables)

Low-Sodium Beef Stew (with kidney-safe veggies)

Grilled Shrimp Skewers with Zucchini

Vegetable Stir-Fry (with tofu, kidney-friendly veggies, low-sodium soy alternative)

Slow-Cooker Chicken and Veggies (kidney-safe, low-sodium broth)

Kidney-Safe Mushroom Risotto (using low-sodium broth)

Herb-Roasted Chicken with Quinoa

Low Sodium | Mid-Protein | Heart-Healthy

🍽 Servings: 2

⏱ Prep Time: 10 minutes

🔍 Cook Time: 25 minutes

Ingredients

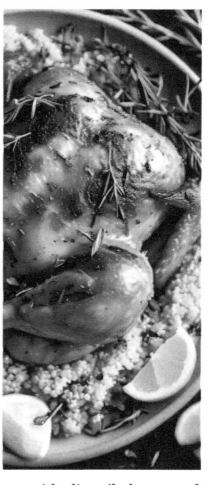

- 2 small chicken breasts
- 1/2 cup quinoa, rinsed
- 1 cup low-sodium chicken broth
- 1 tbsp olive oil
- 1 tsp dried thyme
- 1 tsp dried rosemary
- Fresh parsley for garnish

Directions

1. Preheat the oven to 375°F (190°C). Rub the chicken breasts with olive oil, thyme, and rosemary.
2. Roast the chicken for 20-25 minutes, or until cooked through.

3. Meanwhile, cook quinoa in low-sodium chicken broth according to package instructions (about 15 minutes).
4. Serve the herb-roasted chicken on a bed of quinoa, garnished with fresh parsley.

Nutritional Info Per Serving:

Calories: 290 | Protein: 26g | Carbs: 24g | Sodium: 90mg | Cholesterol: 50mg | Potassium: 220mg | Phosphorus: 200mg

Grilled Salmon with Steamed Asparagus

Low Sodium | Low Potassium | High Protein

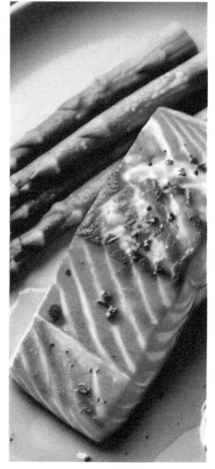

Servings: 2

Prep Time: 10 minutes

Cook Time: 15 minutes

Ingredients

- 2 small salmon fillets
- 1/2 bunch asparagus, trimmed
- 1 tbsp olive oil
- 1 tbsp lemon juice
- Fresh dill for garnish

Directions

- Preheat the grill to medium heat. Brush the salmon fillets with olive oil and grill for 5-7 minutes on each side until cooked through.
- Steam the asparagus for 4-5 minutes until tender.

- Drizzle the salmon and asparagus with lemon juice and garnish with fresh dill before serving.

Nutritional Info Per Serving:

Calories: 280 | Protein: 24g | Carbs: 8g | Sodium: 60mg | Cholesterol: 60mg | Potassium: 260mg | Phosphorus: 230mg

Baked Chicken Thighs with Roasted Carrots

Low Sodium | Low Potassium | Mid-Protein

🍴 Servings: 2

⏱ Prep Time: 10 minutes

🔍 Cook Time: 30 minutes

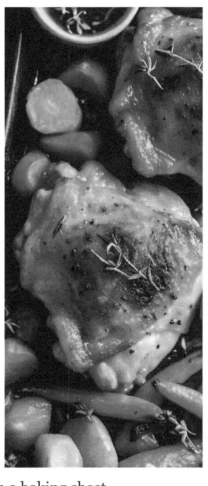

Ingredients

- 2 chicken thighs (skinless)
- 1/2 lb carrots, sliced
- 1 tbsp olive oil
- 1 tsp dried thyme
- 1 tsp garlic powder
- Fresh parsley for garnish

Directions

1. Preheat the oven to 375°F (190°C). Toss the carrots with olive oil, thyme, and garlic powder, and spread on a baking sheet.
2. Place the chicken thighs on the baking sheet and roast for 25-30 minutes until cooked through.

3. Serve the chicken thighs with roasted carrots, garnished with fresh parsley.

Nutritional Info Per Serving:

Calories: 320 | Protein: 26g | Carbs: 18g | Sodium: 80mg | Cholesterol: 80mg | Potassium: 250mg | Phosphorus: 210mg

Turkey Meatballs with Kidney-Safe Tomato Sauce

Low Sodium | Low Potassium | High Protein

🍴 Servings: 2

⏱ Prep Time: 15 minutes

🔍 Cook Time: 25 minutes

Ingredients

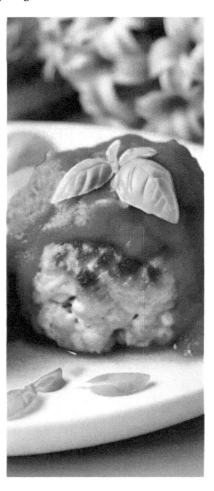

- 1/2 lb ground turkey (lean)
- 1/4 cup breadcrumbs (low-sodium)
- 1 egg white
- 1/2 tsp garlic powder
- 1/2 cup kidney-safe tomato sauce (low potassium, low sodium)
- 1 tbsp olive oil
- Fresh basil for garnish

Directions

1. Preheat the oven to 375°F (190°C). In a bowl, mix ground turkey, breadcrumbs, egg white, and garlic powder.

2. Form the mixture into small meatballs and place on a baking sheet.
3. Bake for 20-25 minutes until cooked through.
4. Heat the tomato sauce in a small saucepan. Serve the meatballs topped with sauce and garnish with fresh basil.

Nutritional Info Per Serving:

Calories: 260 | Protein: 25g | Carbs: 14g | Sodium: 120mg | Cholesterol: 50mg | Potassium: 190mg | Phosphorus: 180mg

Pork Tenderloin with Steamed Broccoli

Low Sodium | Low Potassium | High Protein

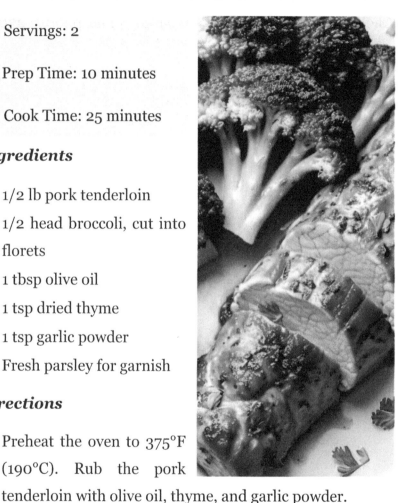

🍴 Servings: 2

⏱ Prep Time: 10 minutes

🔍 Cook Time: 25 minutes

Ingredients

- 1/2 lb pork tenderloin
- 1/2 head broccoli, cut into florets
- 1 tbsp olive oil
- 1 tsp dried thyme
- 1 tsp garlic powder
- Fresh parsley for garnish

Directions

1. Preheat the oven to 375°F (190°C). Rub the pork tenderloin with olive oil, thyme, and garlic powder.
2. Roast the pork for 20-25 minutes, or until cooked through.
3. Steam the broccoli florets for 4-5 minutes until tender.
4. Serve the pork with steamed broccoli and garnish with fresh parsley.

Nutritional Info Per Serving:

Calories: 250 | Protein: 28g | Carbs: 10g | Sodium: 70mg | Cholesterol: 70mg | Potassium: 240mg | Phosphorus: 220mg

Grilled Tilapia with Lemon and Quinoa

Low Sodium | Low Potassium | High Protein

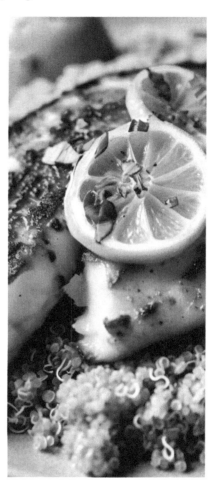

🍽 Servings: 2

⏱ Prep Time: 10 minutes

🔍 Cook Time: 20 minutes

Ingredients

- 2 small tilapia fillets
- 1/2 cup quinoa, rinsed
- 1 cup low-sodium vegetable broth
- 1 tbsp olive oil
- 1 tbsp lemon juice
- Fresh parsley for garnish

Directions

1. Grill the tilapia fillets for 5-7 minutes on each side until cooked through.
2. In a small saucepan, bring vegetable broth to a boil and add quinoa. Cover and cook for 15 minutes until tender.
3. Drizzle the grilled tilapia with lemon juice and serve with quinoa, garnished with fresh parsley.

Nutritional Info Per Serving:

Calories: 270 | Protein: 24g | Carbs: 26g | Sodium: 80mg |
Cholesterol: 50mg | Potassium: 200mg | Phosphorus: 220mg

Low-Sodium Chicken Stir-Fry with Brown Rice

Low Sodium | Mid-Protein | High Fiber

🔖 Servings: 2

⏱ Prep Time: 10 minutes

🔍 Cook Time: 20 minutes

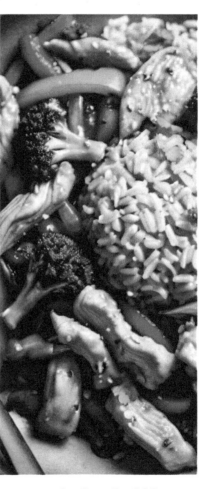

Ingredients

- 1 small chicken breast, sliced
- 1/2 cup brown rice, rinsed
- 1/4 cup sliced bell peppers
- 1/4 cup sliced zucchini
- 1 tsp olive oil
- 1 tbsp low-sodium soy sauce alternative
- Fresh parsley for garnish

Directions

1. In a small saucepan, bring water to a boil and add brown rice. Cook for 15 minutes until tender.

2. Heat olive oil in a large skillet and add chicken slices. Cook for 5-7 minutes until browned.

3. Add the bell peppers and zucchini to the skillet and stir-fry for an additional 5 minutes.

4. Stir in the low-sodium soy sauce alternative and serve over brown rice, garnished with parsley.

Nutritional Info Per Serving:

Calories: 280 | Protein: 22g | Carbs: 34g | Sodium: 120mg | Cholesterol: 40mg | Potassium: 220mg | Phosphorus: 200mg

Kidney-Friendly Shepherd's Pie (using Lean Ground Beef, No-Salt Mashed Cauliflower)

Low Sodium | Mid-Protein | Heart-Healthy

🍽 Servings: 2

⏱ Prep Time: 15 minutes

🔍 Cook Time: 30 minutes

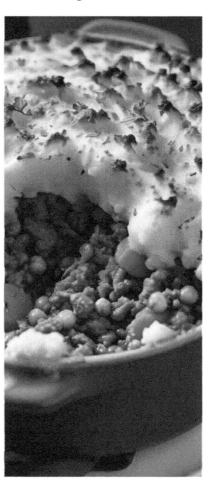

Ingredients

- 1/2 lb lean ground beef
- 1/2 cup kidney-friendly vegetables (carrots, zucchini)
- 1/2 head cauliflower, steamed and mashed
- 1 tbsp olive oil
- 1/2 tsp garlic powder
- Fresh parsley for garnish

Directions

1. Preheat the oven to 375°F (190°C). In a skillet, brown the ground beef over medium heat, breaking it up as it cooks.

2. Add the kidney-friendly vegetables and cook for 5-7 minutes until tender.

3. Spread the cooked beef and veggies in an oven-safe dish. Top with mashed cauliflower mixed with olive oil and garlic powder.

4. Bake for 20 minutes until the top is golden. Garnish with fresh parsley and serve.

Nutritional Info Per Serving:

Calories: 300 | Protein: 22g | Carbs: 18g | Sodium: 80mg | Cholesterol: 60mg | Potassium: 260mg | Phosphorus: 220mg

Baked Cod with Roasted Zucchini and Brown Rice

Low Sodium | Low Potassium | High Protein

🍽 Servings: 2

⏱ Prep Time: 10 minutes

🔍 Cook Time: 25 minutes

Ingredients

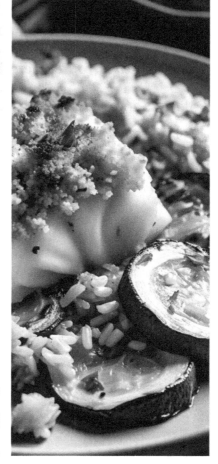

- 2 small cod fillets
- 1/2 cup brown rice, rinsed
- 1/2 cup diced zucchini
- 1 tbsp olive oil
- 1 tbsp lemon juice
- Fresh dill for garnish

Directions

1. Preheat the oven to 375°F (190°C). Place the cod fillets on a baking sheet, drizzle with olive oil, and bake for 15-20 minutes until cooked through.

2. In a saucepan, bring water to a boil, add brown rice, and cook for 15 minutes until tender.
3. Toss the diced zucchini with olive oil and roast for 10 minutes until tender.
4. Serve the baked cod with roasted zucchini and brown rice, garnished with fresh dill and lemon juice.

Nutritional Info Per Serving:

Calories: 260 | Protein: 22g | Carbs: 28g | Sodium: 90mg | Cholesterol: 50mg | Potassium: 230mg | Phosphorus: 200mg

Kidney-Friendly Veggie Pizza (using Low-Potassium Sauce, Kidney-Safe Veggies)

Low Sodium | Low Potassium | High Fiber

🍽 Servings: 2

⏱ Prep Time: 15 minutes

🔍 Cook Time: 20 minutes

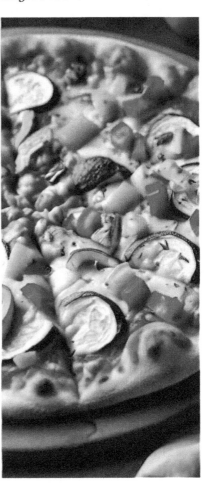

Ingredients

- 1 small whole wheat pizza crust (low sodium)
- 1/4 cup low-potassium tomato sauce
- 1/4 cup shredded mozzarella (low sodium)
- 1/4 cup diced bell peppers
- 1/4 cup sliced zucchini
- Fresh basil for garnish

Directions

1. Preheat the oven to 400°F (200°C). Spread the low-potassium tomato sauce over the pizza crust.

2. Top with shredded mozzarella, diced bell peppers, and zucchini slices.

3. Bake for 15-20 minutes until the cheese is melted and bubbly.

4. Garnish with fresh basil and serve immediately.

Nutritional Info Per Serving:

Calories: 300 | Protein: 12g | Carbs: 42g | Sodium: 140mg | Cholesterol: 15mg | Potassium: 160mg | Phosphorus: 150mg

Grilled Chicken with Couscous and Roasted Red Peppers

Low Sodium | Mid-Protein | Heart-Healthy

🍽 Servings: 2

⏱ Prep Time: 10 minutes

🔍 Cook Time: 20 minutes

Ingredients

- 1 small chicken breast, grilled and sliced
- 1/2 cup couscous, rinsed
- 1/4 cup roasted red peppers
- 1 tbsp olive oil
- 1 tsp lemon juice
- Fresh parsley for garnish

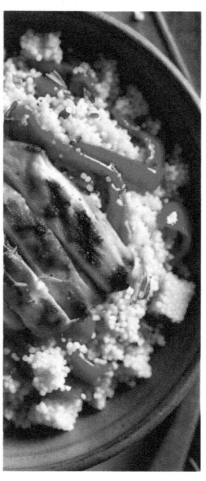

Directions

1. Preheat the grill to medium heat and grill the chicken breast for 5-7 minutes on each side until cooked through.

2. In a small saucepan, bring water to a boil and add couscous. Cover and let sit for 5 minutes.

3. Stir in the roasted red peppers, olive oil, and lemon juice.

4. Serve the grilled chicken with couscous, garnished with fresh parsley.

Nutritional Info Per Serving:

Calories: 280 | Protein: 24g | Carbs: 28g | Sodium: 90mg | Cholesterol: 40mg | Potassium: 180mg | Phosphorus: 170mg

Stuffed Bell Peppers (with Lean Turkey, Brown Rice)

Low Sodium | Mid-Protein | High Fiber

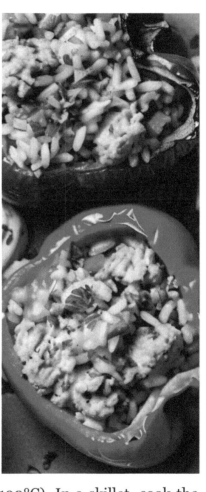

 Servings: 2

 Prep Time: 10 minutes

 Cook Time: 25 minutes

Ingredients

- 2 large bell peppers, tops removed and seeds discarded
- 1/2 lb lean ground turkey
- 1/4 cup cooked brown rice
- 1/4 cup kidney-safe tomato sauce (low sodium)
- 1 tbsp olive oil
- Fresh parsley for garnish

Directions

1. Preheat the oven to 375°F (190°C). In a skillet, cook the ground turkey for 5-7 minutes until browned.
2. Mix the cooked turkey with brown rice and tomato sauce.

3. Stuff the bell peppers with the turkey mixture and place them in an oven-safe dish.
4. Bake for 20-25 minutes until the peppers are tender. Garnish with fresh parsley and serve.

Nutritional Info Per Serving:

Calories: 260 | Protein: 20g | Carbs: 24g | Sodium: 120mg | Cholesterol: 50mg | Potassium: 220mg | Phosphorus: 180mg

Grilled Turkey Burgers (Low-Sodium, Served with a Side of Mixed Greens)

Low Sodium | Mid-Protein | Heart-Healthy

🍴 Servings: 2

⏱ Prep Time: 10 minutes

🔍 Cook Time: 10 minutes

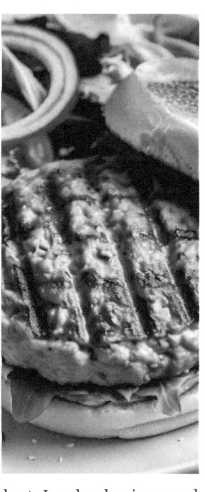

Ingredients

- 1/2 lb ground turkey (lean)
- 1/4 cup breadcrumbs (low sodium)
- 1 egg white
- 1 tsp garlic powder
- 2 low-sodium whole wheat burger buns
- 2 cups mixed greens
- 1 tbsp olive oil for dressing

Directions

1. Preheat the grill to medium heat. In a bowl, mix ground turkey, breadcrumbs, egg white, and garlic powder.

2. Form the mixture into two patties and grill for 5-7 minutes on each side until cooked through.

3. Serve the turkey burgers on whole wheat buns with a side of mixed greens drizzled with olive oil.

Nutritional Info Per Serving:

Calories: 320 | Protein: 22g | Carbs: 34g | Sodium: 130mg | Cholesterol: 50mg | Potassium: 180mg | Phosphorus: 160mg

Baked Lemon Herb Chicken with Steamed Carrots

Low Sodium | Low Potassium | Mid-Protein

🍽 Servings: 2

⏲ Prep Time: 10 minutes

🔍 Cook Time: 25 minutes

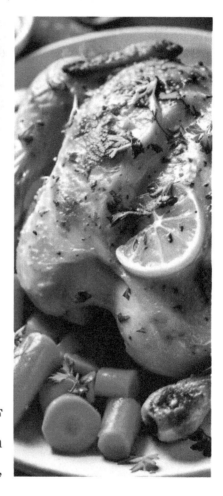

Ingredients

- 2 small chicken breasts
- 1/2 lb carrots, sliced
- 1 tbsp olive oil
- 1 tbsp lemon juice
- 1 tsp dried rosemary
- Fresh parsley for garnish

Directions

1. Preheat the oven to 375°F (190°C). Rub the chicken breasts with olive oil, lemon juice, and rosemary.
2. Bake the chicken for 20-25 minutes until cooked through.
3. Steam the sliced carrots for 4-5 minutes until tender.

4. Serve the baked chicken with steamed carrots, garnished with fresh parsley.

Nutritional Info Per Serving:

Calories: 280 | Protein: 26g | Carbs: 14g | Sodium: 70mg | Cholesterol: 50mg | Potassium: 240mg | Phosphorus: 200mg

Chicken and Rice Casserole (Low-Sodium Version with Kidney-Friendly Vegetables)

Low Sodium | Mid-Protein | Heart-Healthy

🍽 Servings: 2

⏱ Prep Time: 10 minutes

🔍 Cook Time: 30 minutes

Ingredients

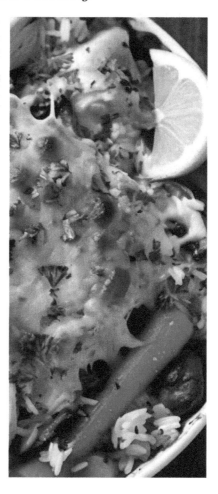

- 1 small chicken breast, diced
- 1/2 cup brown rice, rinsed
- 1/2 cup kidney-safe vegetables (e.g., carrots, zucchini)
- 1 cup low-sodium chicken broth
- 1 tbsp olive oil
- Fresh parsley for garnish

Directions

1. Preheat the oven to 350°F (175°C). In a skillet, cook the diced chicken for 5 minutes until browned.
2. In an oven-safe dish, mix the cooked chicken, brown rice, vegetables, and chicken broth.
3. Cover with foil and bake for 25-30 minutes until the rice is tender.
4. Garnish with fresh parsley before serving.

Nutritional Info Per Serving:

Calories: 320 | Protein: 22g | Carbs: 30g | Sodium: 100mg | Cholesterol: 45mg | Potassium: 240mg | Phosphorus: 200mg

Low-Sodium Beef Stew (with Kidney-Safe Veggies)

Low Sodium | Mid-Protein | High Fiber

🍴 Servings: 2

⏱ Prep Time: 15 minutes

🔍 Cook Time: 40 minutes

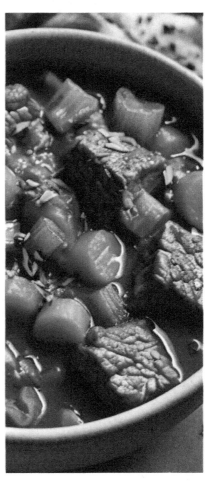

Ingredients

- 1/2 lb lean beef, cubed
- 1 cup low-sodium beef broth
- 1/2 cup diced carrots
- 1/2 cup diced celery
- 1/4 cup diced onions
- 1 tbsp olive oil
- Fresh parsley for garnish

Directions

- In a large pot, heat olive oil over medium heat and brown the beef cubes for 5-7 minutes.

- Add diced carrots, celery, and onions to the pot and cook for another 5 minutes.
- Pour in the low-sodium beef broth, cover, and simmer for 30 minutes until the beef is tender.
- Garnish with fresh parsley and serve warm.

Nutritional Info Per Serving:

Calories: 290 | Protein: 24g | Carbs: 18g | Sodium: 120mg | Cholesterol: 70mg | Potassium: 220mg | Phosphorus: 190mg

Grilled Shrimp Skewers with Zucchini

Low Sodium | Low Potassium | High Protein

🍽 Servings: 2

⏱ Prep Time: 10 minutes

🔍 Cook Time: 10 minutes

Ingredients

- 1/2 lb shrimp, peeled and deveined
- 1/2 cup zucchini slices
- 1 tbsp olive oil
- 1 tbsp lemon juice
- 1 tsp garlic powder
- Fresh parsley for garnish

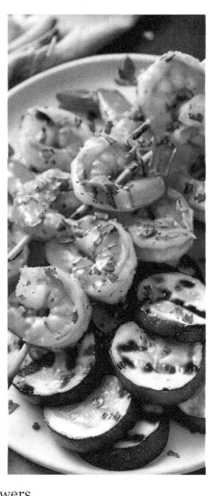

Directions

1. Preheat the grill to medium heat. Thread the shrimp and zucchini slices onto skewers.
2. In a small bowl, mix olive oil, lemon juice, and garlic powder. Brush the shrimp and zucchini with the mixture.
3. Grill for 3-4 minutes on each side until the shrimp is cooked through.

4. Garnish with fresh parsley and serve immediately.

Nutritional Info Per Serving:

Calories: 220 | Protein: 25g | Carbs: 8g | Sodium: 80mg | Cholesterol: 170mg | Potassium: 180mg | Phosphorus: 180mg

Vegetable Stir-Fry (with Tofu, Kidney-Friendly Veggies, Low-Sodium Soy Alternative)

Low Sodium | Low Potassium | Vegan

🍽 Servings: 2

⏱ Prep Time: 10 minutes

🔍 Cook Time: 10 minutes

Ingredients

- 1/2 block firm tofu, cubed
- 1/2 cup sliced zucchini
- 1/4 cup sliced bell peppers
- 1/4 cup sliced carrots
- 1 tbsp olive oil
- 1 tbsp low-sodium soy sauce alternative
- Fresh parsley for garnish

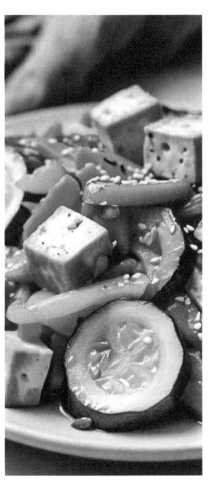

Directions

1. Heat olive oil in a non-stick skillet over medium heat. Add the cubed tofu and cook for 5 minutes until lightly browned.

2. Add the zucchini, bell peppers, and carrots to the skillet. Stir-fry for another 5-7 minutes until the vegetables are tender.
3. Stir in the low-sodium soy sauce alternative and cook for 1 more minute.
4. Garnish with fresh parsley and serve warm.

Nutritional Info Per Serving:

Calories: 190 | Protein: 12g | Carbs: 14g | Sodium: 80mg | Cholesterol: 0mg | Potassium: 160mg | Phosphorus: 110mg

Slow-Cooker Chicken and Veggies (Kidney-Safe, Low-Sodium Broth)

Low Sodium | Mid-Protein | Heart-Healthy

🍽 Servings: 2

⏱ Prep Time: 10 minutes

🔍 Cook Time: 4 hours (slow cooker)

Ingredients

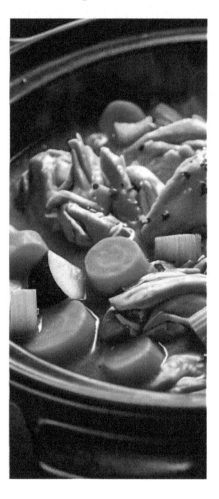

- 1 small chicken breast, diced
- 1 cup low-sodium chicken broth
- 1/4 cup diced carrots
- 1/4 cup diced celery
- 1/4 cup diced zucchini
- 1 tsp olive oil
- Fresh parsley for garnish

Directions

1. Add diced chicken, vegetables, and low-sodium chicken broth to the slow cooker.

2. Cook on low for 4 hours, or until the chicken is tender and the vegetables are cooked.

3. Serve hot, garnished with fresh parsley.

Nutritional Info Per Serving:

Calories: 230 | Protein: 22g | Carbs: 16g | Sodium: 90mg | Cholesterol: 45mg | Potassium: 220mg | Phosphorus: 190mg

Kidney-Safe Mushroom Risotto (using Low-Sodium Broth)

Low Sodium | Low Potassium | High Fiber

🍴 Servings: 2

⏲ Prep Time: 10 minutes

🔍 Cook Time: 20 minutes

Ingredients

- 1/2 cup Arborio rice
- 1 cup low-sodium vegetable broth
- 1/2 cup sliced mushrooms (low potassium)
- 1 tbsp olive oil
- 1/2 tsp garlic powder
- Fresh parsley for garnish

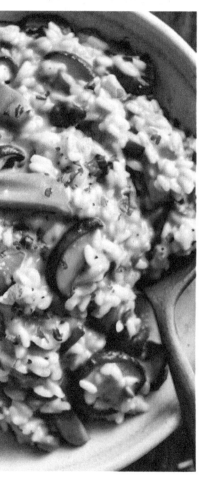

Directions

1. In a large skillet, heat olive oil over medium heat and sauté the sliced mushrooms for 3-4 minutes.

2. Add the Arborio rice and cook for 1 minute, stirring frequently.

3. Gradually add the low-sodium vegetable broth, 1/4 cup at a time, stirring constantly. Allow each addition of broth to be absorbed before adding more.

4. Continue adding broth and stirring for about 15-20 minutes until the rice is tender and creamy.

5. Garnish with fresh parsley and serve warm.

Nutritional Info Per Serving:

Calories: 240 | Protein: 5g | Carbs: 40g | Sodium: 60mg | Cholesterol: 0mg | Potassium: 140mg | Phosphorus: 100mg

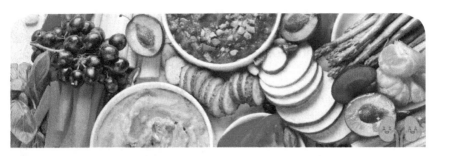

CHAPTER 8: SNACK IDEAS FOR STAGE 3 CKD

Sliced Apples with Almond Butter

Carrot and Cucumber Sticks with Hummus (low-sodium)

Unsalted Rice Cakes with Peanut Butter

Air-Popped Popcorn with Olive Oil and Herbs

Low-Sodium Cheese and Whole Grain Crackers

Sliced Bell Peppers with Low-Sodium Cream Cheese

Homemade Low-Sodium Trail Mix (unsalted nuts, dried cranberries)

Cucumber Slices with Lemon and Olive Oil

Fresh Pear Slices with Almonds

Low-Sodium Rice Crackers with Hummus

Sliced Apples with Almond Butter

Low Sodium | Low Potassium | Heart-Healthy

🍽 Servings: 2

⏱ Prep Time: 5 minutes

🔍 Cook Time: None

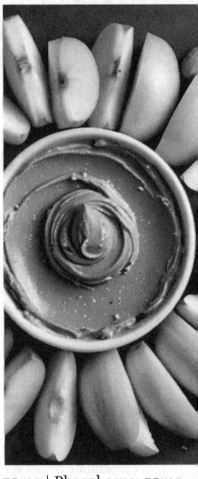

Ingredients

- 1 medium apple, thinly sliced
- 2 tbsp almond butter (unsalted, natural)

Directions

1. Slice the apple into thin wedges.
2. Divide the almond butter between two servings and serve alongside the apple slices for dipping.

Nutritional Info Per Serving:

Calories: 160 | Protein: 4g | Carbs: 24g | Sodium: 0mg | Cholesterol: 0mg | Potassium: 150mg | Phosphorus: 50mg

Carrot and Cucumber Sticks with Hummus (Low-Sodium)

Low Sodium | Low Potassium | High Fiber

🍽 Servings: 2

⏱ Prep Time: 5 minutes

🔍 Cook Time: None

Ingredients

- 1 medium carrot, cut into sticks
- 1/2 cucumber, sliced into sticks
- 1/4 cup low-sodium hummus

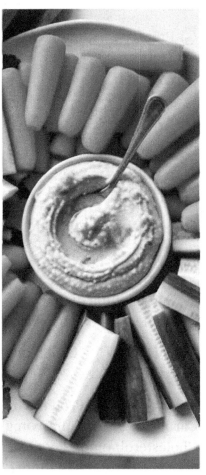

Directions

- Arrange the carrot and cucumber sticks on a plate.
- Serve with hummus for dipping.

Nutritional Info Per Serving:

Calories: 90 | Protein: 3g | Carbs: 14g | Sodium: 40mg | Cholesterol: 0mg | Potassium: 180mg | Phosphorus: 40mg

Unsalted Rice Cakes with Peanut Butter

Low Sodium | Low Potassium | Heart-Healthy

🍽 Servings: 2

⏱ Prep Time: 5 minutes

🔍 Cook Time: None

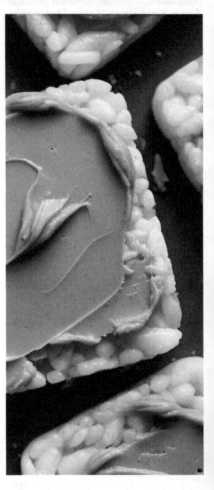

Ingredients

- 2 unsalted rice cakes
- 2 tbsp peanut butter (unsalted, natural)

Directions

1. Spread peanut butter evenly on each rice cake.
2. Serve immediately as a crunchy, satisfying snack.

Nutritional Info Per Serving:

Calories: 180 | Protein: 6g | Carbs: 24g | Sodium: 0mg | Cholesterol: 0mg | Potassium: 160mg | Phosphorus: 60mg

Air-Popped Popcorn with Olive Oil and Herbs

Low Sodium | Low Potassium | High Fiber

🍽 Servings: 2

⏱ Prep Time: 5 minutes

🔍 Cook Time: 5 minutes

Ingredients

- 1/4 cup popcorn kernels (air-popped)
- 1 tbsp olive oil
- 1/2 tsp dried rosemary or thyme

Directions

1. Air-pop the popcorn kernels according to the manufacturer's instructions.
2. Drizzle with olive oil and sprinkle with herbs.
3. Toss well and serve immediately.

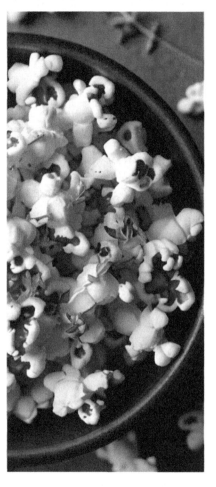

Nutritional Info Per Serving:

Calories: 120 | Protein: 2g | Carbs: 18g | Sodium: 0mg | Cholesterol: 0mg | Potassium: 60mg | Phosphorus: 40mg

Low-Sodium Cheese and Whole Grain Crackers

Low Sodium | Low Potassium | Mid-Protein

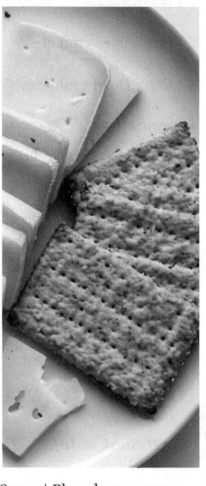

🍽 Servings: 2

⏱ Prep Time: 2 minutes

🔍 Cook Time: None

Ingredients

- 2 oz low-sodium cheese
- 8 whole grain crackers (low sodium)

Directions

1. Slice the cheese into small squares and arrange alongside the crackers.
2. Serve as a simple, kidney-safe snack.

Nutritional Info Per Serving:

Calories: 150 | Protein: 6g | Carbs: 18g | Sodium: 100mg | Cholesterol: 10mg | Potassium: 80mg | Phosphorus: 70mg

Sliced Bell Peppers with Low-Sodium Cream Cheese

Low Sodium | Low Potassium | Heart-Healthy

🍽 Servings: 2

⏱ Prep Time: 5 minutes

🔍 Cook Time: None

Ingredients

- 1/2 large bell pepper, sliced
- 2 tbsp low-sodium cream cheese

Directions

1. Spread low-sodium cream cheese onto bell pepper slices.
2. Serve as a refreshing and crunchy snack.

Nutritional Info Per Serving:

Calories: 80 | Protein: 3g | Carbs: 6g | Sodium: 40mg | Cholesterol: 5mg | Potassium: 120mg | Phosphorus: 40mg

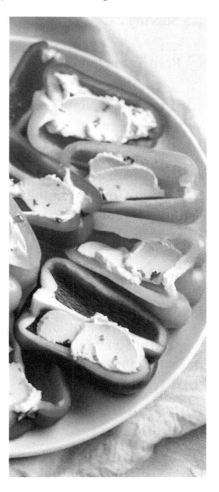

Homemade Low-Sodium Trail Mix (Unsalted Nuts, Dried Cranberries)

Low Sodium | Low Potassium | Heart-Healthy

🍽 Servings: 2

⏱ Prep Time: 5 minutes

🔍 Cook Time: None

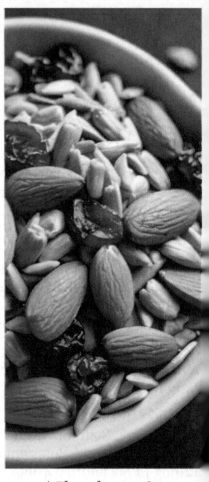

Ingredients

- 1/4 cup unsalted almonds
- 1/4 cup dried cranberries (unsweetened)
- 1/4 cup unsalted sunflower seeds

Directions

1. Combine the almonds, cranberries, and sunflower seeds in a small bowl.
2. Serve immediately or store for later.

Nutritional Info Per Serving:

Calories: 170 | Protein: 5g | Carbs: 18g | Sodium: 5mg | Cholesterol: 0mg | Potassium: 120mg | Phosphorus: 80mg

Cucumber Slices with Lemon and Olive Oil

Low Sodium | Low Potassium | Refreshing

🍽 Servings: 2

⏱ Prep Time: 5 minutes

🔍 Cook Time: None

Ingredients

- 1/2 cucumber, thinly sliced
- 1 tbsp olive oil
- 1 tsp lemon juice
- Fresh parsley for garnish

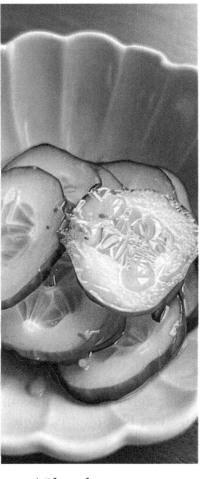

Directions

1. Arrange the cucumber slices on a plate.
2. Drizzle with olive oil and lemon juice.
3. Garnish with fresh parsley and serve immediately.

Nutritional Info Per Serving:

Calories: 80 | Protein: 1g | Carbs: 5g | Sodium: 0mg | Cholesterol: 0mg | Potassium: 60mg | Phosphorus: 10mg

Fresh Pear Slices with Almonds

Low Sodium | Low Potassium | High Fiber

🍴 Servings: 2

⏱ Prep Time: 5 minutes

🔍 Cook Time: None

Ingredients

- 1 small pear, sliced
- 1/4 cup unsalted almonds

Directions

- Slice the pear into thin wedges.
- Serve alongside the almonds for a light and satisfying snack.

Nutritional Info Per Serving:

Calories: 150 | Protein: 4g | Carbs: 20g | Sodium: 0mg | Cholesterol: 0mg | Potassium: 100mg | Phosphorus: 40mg

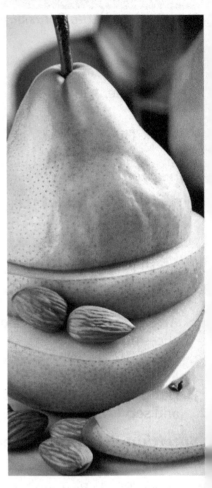

Low-Sodium Rice Crackers with Hummus

Low Sodium | Low Potassium | High Fiber

🍴 Servings: 2

⏱ Prep Time: 5 minutes

🔍 Cook Time: None

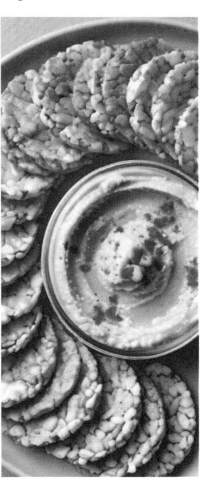

Ingredients

- 8 low-sodium rice crackers
- 1/4 cup low-sodium hummus

Directions

- Serve the rice crackers with hummus for dipping.

Nutritional Info Per Serving:

Calories: 120 | Protein: 3g | Carbs: 18g | Sodium: 40mg | Cholesterol: 0mg | Potassium: 50mg | Phosphorus: 30mg

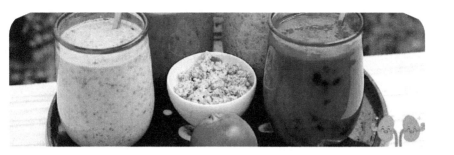

CHAPTER 9: SMOOTHIES AND BEVERAGES FOR STAGE 3 CKD

Strawberry-Pineapple Smoothie (with almond milk)

Blueberry-Apple Smoothie (using low-potassium fruits)

Cucumber-Melon Smoothie (hydrating and low-potassium)

Cranberry-Pear Smoothie (with almond milk)

Mixed Berry Smoothie (strawberries, raspberries, and almond milk)

Mango-Cucumber Smoothie (light and refreshing, low potassium)

Grape-Peach Smoothie (kidney-friendly fruit blend)

Watermelon-Basil Smoothie (hydrating and low-sodium)

Apple-Cinnamon Smoothie (with almond or coconut milk)

Low-Sodium Herbal Tea (iced or hot)

Strawberry-Pineapple Smoothie (with Almond Milk)

Low Sodium | Low Potassium | Dairy-Free

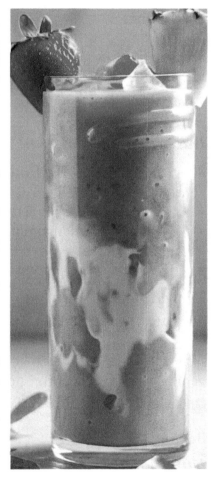

🍽 Servings: 2

⏱ Prep Time: 5 minutes

🔍 Cook Time: None

Ingredients

- 1/2 cup fresh or frozen strawberries
- 1/2 cup fresh or frozen pineapple chunks
- 1 cup unsweetened almond milk
- 1 tsp honey or maple syrup (optional)

Directions

1. In a blender, combine strawberries, pineapple, and almond milk.
2. Blend until smooth and creamy.
3. Serve immediately, with a drizzle of honey if desired.

Nutritional Info Per Serving:

Calories: 120 | Protein: 2g | Carbs: 24g | Sodium: 30mg | Cholesterol: 0mg | Potassium: 120mg | Phosphorus: 40mg

Blueberry-Apple Smoothie (Using Low-Potassium Fruits)

Low Potassium | Low Sodium | High Fiber

🍽 Servings: 2

⏱ Prep Time: 5 minutes

🔍 Cook Time: None

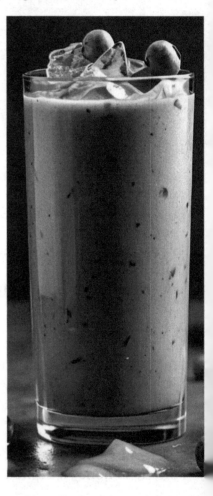

Ingredients

- 1/2 cup fresh or frozen blueberries
- 1/2 small apple, chopped
- 1 cup unsweetened almond milk
- 1 tbsp chia seeds (optional)

Directions

1. In a blender, combine blueberries, apple, and almond milk.
2. Blend until smooth. Add chia seeds for extra fiber, if desired.
3. Serve immediately.

Nutritional Info Per Serving:

Calories: 110 | Protein: 2g | Carbs: 22g | Sodium: 25mg | Cholesterol: 0mg | Potassium: 100mg | Phosphorus: 40mg

Cucumber-Melon Smoothie (Hydrating and Low-Potassium)

Low Potassium | Low Sodium | Hydrating

Servings: 2

Prep Time: 5 minutes

Cook Time: None

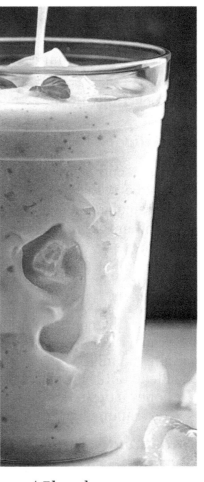

Ingredients

- 1/2 cup diced cucumber
- 1/2 cup diced honeydew melon
- 1/2 cup ice cubes
- 1 cup water

Directions

1. In a blender, combine cucumber, melon, and ice.
2. Add water and blend until smooth and refreshing.
3. Serve immediately.

Nutritional Info Per Serving:

Calories: 60 | Protein: 1g | Carbs: 15g | Sodium: 10mg | Cholesterol: 0mg | Potassium: 70mg | Phosphorus: 10mg

Cranberry-Pear Smoothie (with Almond Milk)

Low Potassium | Low Sodium | Heart-Healthy

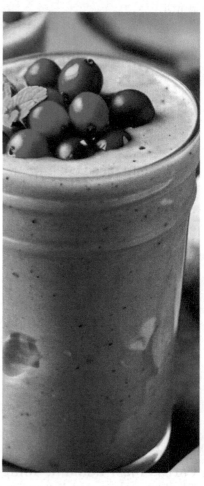

📇 Servings: 2

⏱ Prep Time: 5 minutes

🔍 Cook Time: None

Ingredients

- 1/4 cup unsweetened cranberry juice
- 1/2 small pear, chopped
- 1 cup unsweetened almond milk
- 1 tsp honey (optional)

Directions

1. In a blender, combine cranberry juice, pear, and almond milk.
2. Blend until smooth, adding honey if desired.
3. Serve immediately.

Nutritional Info Per Serving:

Calories: 80 | Protein: 2g | Carbs: 18g | Sodium: 20mg | Cholesterol: 0mg | Potassium: 80mg | Phosphorus: 30mg

Mixed Berry Smoothie (Strawberries, Raspberries, and Almond Milk)

Low Sodium | Low Potassium | Dairy-Free

🎞 Servings: 2

⏱ Prep Time: 5 minutes

🔍 Cook Time: None

Ingredients

- 1/4 cup fresh or frozen strawberries
- 1/4 cup fresh or frozen raspberries
- 1 cup unsweetened almond milk
- 1 tsp honey or maple syrup (optional)

Directions

1. In a blender, combine strawberries, raspberries, and almond milk.
2. Blend until smooth and creamy.
3. Serve immediately with a drizzle of honey, if desired.

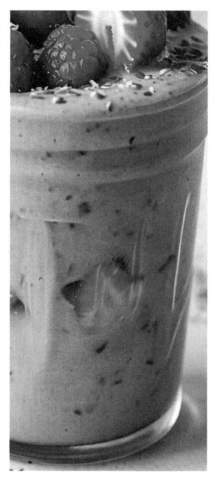

Nutritional Info Per Serving:

Calories: 110 | Protein: 2g | Carbs: 22g | Sodium: 30mg | Cholesterol: 0mg | Potassium: 100mg | Phosphorus: 40mg

Mango-Cucumber Smoothie (Light and Refreshing, Low Potassium)

Low Sodium | Low Potassium | Refreshing

🍽 Servings: 2

⏱ Prep Time: 5 minutes

🔍 Cook Time: None

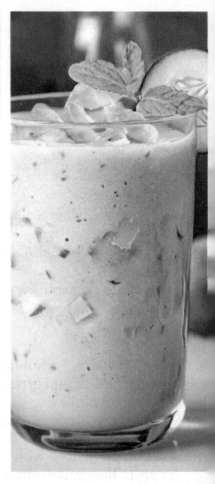

Ingredients

- 1/2 cup fresh or frozen mango
- 1/4 cup diced cucumber
- 1 cup water
- 1 tbsp lemon juice

Directions

1. In a blender, combine mango, cucumber, and water.
2. Add lemon juice and blend until smooth.
3. Serve immediately.

Nutritional Info Per Serving:

Calories: 70 | Protein: 1g | Carbs: 18g | Sodium: 10mg | Cholesterol: 0mg | Potassium: 90mg | Phosphorus: 10mg

Grape-Peach Smoothie (Kidney-Friendly Fruit Blend)

Low Potassium | Low Sodium | Heart-Healthy

🍴 Servings: 2

⏱ Prep Time: 5 minutes

🔍 Cook Time: None

Ingredients

- 1/2 cup seedless grapes
- 1/2 small peach, chopped
- 1 cup unsweetened almond milk
- 1 tsp honey (optional)

Directions

1. In a blender, combine grapes, peach, and almond milk.
2. Blend until smooth, adding honey if desired.
3. Serve immediately.

Nutritional Info Per Serving:

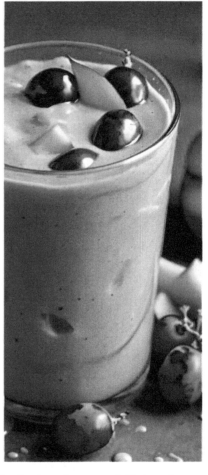

Calories: 90 | Protein: 2g | Carbs: 22g | Sodium: 20mg | Cholesterol: 0mg | Potassium: 80mg | Phosphorus: 30mg

Watermelon-Basil Smoothie (Hydrating and Low-Sodium)

Low Sodium | Low Potassium | Refreshing

🍽 Servings: 2

⏱ Prep Time: 5 minutes

🔍 Cook Time: None

Ingredients

- 1 cup diced watermelon
- 1/4 cup fresh basil leaves
- 1/2 cup ice cubes
- 1/2 cup water

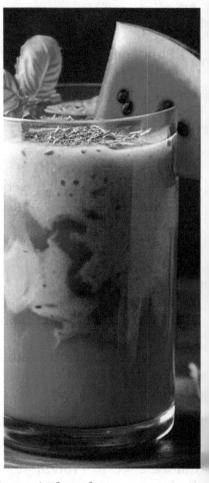

Directions

1. In a blender, combine watermelon, basil, ice, and water.
2. Blend until smooth and refreshing.
3. Serve immediately.

Nutritional Info Per Serving:

Calories: 50 | Protein: 1g | Carbs: 12g | Sodium: 5mg | Cholesterol: 0mg | Potassium: 60mg | Phosphorus: 10mg

Apple-Cinnamon Smoothie (with Almond or Coconut Milk)

Low Sodium | Low Potassium | Dairy-Free

🍴 Servings: 2

⏱ Prep Time: 5 minutes

🔍 Cook Time: None

Ingredients

- 1/2 small apple, chopped
- 1/2 tsp cinnamon
- 1 cup unsweetened almond or coconut milk
- 1 tsp honey or maple syrup (optional)

Directions

1. In a blender, combine apple, cinnamon, and almond or coconut milk.
2. Blend until smooth, adding honey or maple syrup if desired.
3. Serve immediately.

Nutritional Info Per Serving:

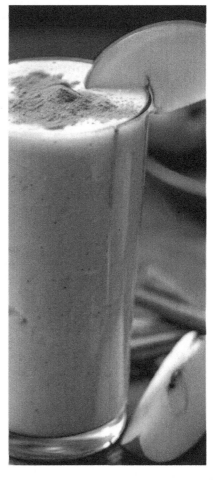

Calories: 100 | Protein: 2g | Carbs: 22g | Sodium: 20mg | Cholesterol: 0mg | Potassium: 80mg | Phosphorus: 30mg

Low-Sodium Herbal Tea (Iced or Hot)

Low Sodium | Caffeine-Free | Refreshing

🍽 Servings: 2

⏱ Prep Time: 2 minutes

🔍 Cook Time: 5 minutes

Ingredients

- 2 cups water
- 2 herbal tea bags (such as peppermint or chamomile)
- Ice cubes (for iced tea)

Directions

1. Boil 2 cups of water and steep the herbal tea bags for 3-5 minutes.
2. Serve hot, or pour over ice for a refreshing iced tea.

Nutritional Info Per Serving:

Calories: 0 | Protein: 0g | Carbs: 0g | Sodium: 0mg | Cholesterol: 0mg | Potassium: 0mg | Phosphorus: 0mg

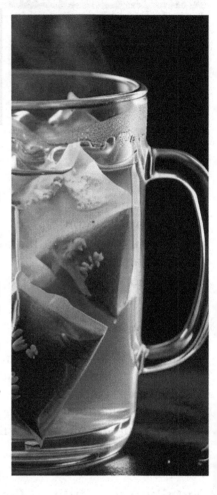

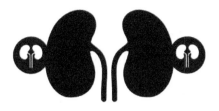

CHAPTER 10: PRACTICAL TIPS FOR DAILY LIVING WITH CKD

Stress-Free Grocery Shopping: A Simple Guide

When it comes to grocery shopping while managing CKD, I know it can feel overwhelming. You've probably spent time squinting at food labels, wondering which foods are safe for your kidneys, and debating whether a particular item should go in your cart. Well, I'm here to take the stress out of the equation. In this section, I'll guide you through simple tips and strategies for navigating the grocery store with confidence, ensuring you're filling your cart with kidney-supportive foods.

1. Start with a Plan

One of the easiest ways to avoid confusion and stress at the store is to start with a well-thought-out plan. Before you head out, take a few minutes to:

- Review your meal plan for the week.
- Write out a grocery list based on the recipes and snacks you plan to make.
- Group similar items together (e.g., fruits and veggies, dairy, proteins) so that you can shop efficiently without wandering back and forth across the aisles.

A printable grocery list template has been included in this cookbook to help you get organized, and trust me, it will make your life a whole lot easier!

2. Master the Art of Food Label Reading

Understanding food labels is one of the most important skills you can develop when managing CKD. There are many things to look out for on a food label, but to keep things simple, here are the three most important things you should look for on labels to ensure your choices are kidney-friendly:

- ✓ **Sodium:** Aim for products that contain less than 140mg of sodium per serving. If you see words like "low sodium," "no added salt," or "sodium-free," those are usually good indicators, but always double-check the actual amount.

✓ **Potassium:** Look for foods labeled "low potassium," or if potassium isn't listed on the label, stick to foods you know are generally low in potassium, like apples, berries, and cucumbers. Avoid items like tomato-based sauces, potatoes, and certain dairy products unless they are marked as low in potassium.

✓ **Phosphorus:** Phosphorus can be tricky since it's not always listed on labels. Keep an eye out for phosphorus additives, such as "phosphate," which are often found in processed and packaged foods. Choose fresh, whole foods when possible.

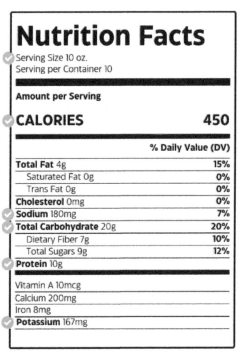

3. Shop the Perimeter of the Store

A simple trick to healthy grocery shopping is to stick to the perimeter of the store. This is where you'll find fresh fruits, vegetables, lean proteins, and unprocessed foods. These items are your best bet when managing CKD since they are naturally lower in sodium, potassium, and phosphorus.

4. Choose Fresh, Frozen, or Low-Sodium Canned Produce

Fresh produce is always a great option, but frozen fruits and vegetables can be just as nutritious—and they last longer! Just make sure to choose options without added salt, sauces, or sugars. If you buy canned vegetables, opt for low-sodium varieties and give them a good rinse before cooking to remove excess salt.

5. Focus on Kidney-Friendly Proteins

Managing your protein intake is key to slowing the progression of CKD. Here are some safe, kidney-friendly protein sources:

- Egg whites
- Skinless chicken breasts
- Lean turkey
- Fresh fish like salmon or tilapia
- Tofu or plant-based protein options

When it comes to meats, always choose fresh over processed and avoid deli meats, bacon, or sausages, as they are typically high in sodium and phosphorus.

6. Opt for Whole Grains

Whole grains like brown rice, quinoa, and whole wheat bread are excellent choices for people with CKD. These foods provide energy without spiking your potassium and phosphorus levels, unlike refined grains. Just be sure to check labels for any hidden sodium.

7. Be Selective with Snacks and Beverages

Snack smart by choosing options like unsalted nuts, rice cakes, and fresh fruit. When it comes to beverages, water should always be your go-to. If you're craving something different, try herbal teas, or infused water with fruits like lemon or berries. Be mindful of drinks high in potassium, such as orange juice, and avoid sugary sodas or sports drinks.

Staying Active and Managing Stress

As someone managing CKD, you've probably heard that staying active and managing stress are two important pillars for maintaining your health. But let's be honest—finding time to exercise and manage stress can feel like another job on top of everything else. That's why I'm here to simplify it for you. In this section, I'll share easy, kidney-safe exercises and stress-relieving techniques that fit seamlessly into your daily routine. No fancy gym equipment, no extreme workouts—just practical ways to stay healthy, both mentally and physically.

1. Low-Impact Exercises for Kidney Health

Physical activity is crucial for maintaining strength, flexibility, and a healthy heart, but not all exercises are suitable for CKD patients. The good news? You don't need high-intensity workouts to see benefits. Here are some simple, low-impact exercises you can incorporate into your routine:

✓ Walking: A brisk 20–30-minute walk around your neighborhood or park can work wonders for your cardiovascular health without putting too much strain on your body. Walking is gentle on your joints and helps to boost circulation.

✓ Swimming or Water Aerobics: If you have access to a pool, swimming is one of the best full-body, low-impact exercises out there. Water supports your body, making it easier on your joints, and you get a great workout without even realizing it.

✓ Yoga: Gentle yoga poses can improve flexibility, strengthen muscles, and help you unwind. There are even specific yoga poses that aid digestion and promote relaxation—two things that are important when managing CKD.

✓ Chair Exercises: For those who might have difficulty standing for long periods, chair exercises are a great option. You can perform simple movements like leg lifts, seated marches, and gentle arm stretches while sitting down.

Consistency is key! Aim for at least 20–30 minutes of physical activity 3–4 times a week. But remember, listen to your body. If you feel fatigued or experience any pain, take a break.

2. The Importance of Managing Stress

Stress is more than just an emotional burden—it can have real physical effects, especially for people managing chronic conditions like CKD. Elevated stress levels can raise your blood pressure and increase the strain on your kidneys, so it's essential to find effective ways to unwind.

Here are a few stress management techniques that you can easily integrate into your daily life:

✓ Deep Breathing: This simple technique can instantly calm your nervous system. *Try the "4-7-8" method:* inhale for 4 seconds, hold your breath for 7 seconds, and exhale slowly for 8 seconds. Repeat this a few times whenever you feel stressed.

- ✓ Meditation: Even just 5 minutes of daily meditation can make a big difference. Sit comfortably, close your eyes, and focus on your breath. Let any thoughts pass without judgment, and gently bring your attention back to your breath.
- ✓ Progressive Muscle Relaxation: This involves tensing and then relaxing different muscle groups in your body, one at a time. Start with your feet and work your way up to your head, releasing tension as you go.
- ✓ Journaling: Writing down your thoughts, worries, and feelings can be a great way to release mental tension. Plus, reflecting on what's been stressing you can sometimes help you find new perspectives or solutions.

3. Combining Movement with Stress Relief

One of the best ways to boost your overall well-being is to combine exercise with stress relief. This could be as simple as going for a nature walk, where you take in the fresh air and focus on the sights and sounds around you. Or perhaps you try yoga, which combines stretching with deep breathing and mindfulness.

By integrating both movement and relaxation into your routine, you're supporting not only your kidneys but your overall mental and physical health. Remember, it's not about perfection—it's about finding small, consistent ways to care for yourself every day.

Quick Meal Prep Ideas for Busy Days

I get it—life gets busy, and the last thing you want to do after a long day is spend hours in the kitchen. But don't worry! With a little bit of planning and some smart meal prep strategies, you can have kidney-friendly meals ready to go, even on your busiest days. In this section, I'll share my favorite quick and easy meal prep ideas to save you time, energy, and stress.

1. Batch Cooking Basics

Batch cooking is a lifesaver for those busy weekdays when you don't have the time or energy to cook from scratch. The idea is simple: prepare larger portions of certain meals, and store them for later. Here's how you can make the most of batch cooking:

- Grain Bowls: Cook a big batch of quinoa, brown rice, or couscous at the start of the week. These grains can serve as the base for several different meals—just add your favorite kidney-friendly protein and veggies for a quick, balanced meal.

- Proteins: Cook up a batch of kidney-friendly proteins like grilled chicken breasts, lean turkey, or baked tofu. Store them in the fridge and add them to salads, sandwiches, or grain bowls throughout the week.

- Roasted Veggies: Roast a tray of vegetables like zucchini, carrots, and bell peppers with a little olive oil and seasoning. You can quickly reheat them for a side dish or toss them into salads and wraps.

2. Freezer-Friendly Meals

If you know you have an extra busy week coming up, freezer meals are a game-changer. Spend a couple of hours over the weekend prepping meals that you can freeze and reheat when needed. Some freezer-friendly, kidney-safe meals include:

- Soups and Stews: Low-sodium chicken soup, lentil soup, or a hearty beef stew are all great options. Simply portion them out into freezer-safe containers, and reheat whenever you need a warm, comforting meal.

- Casseroles: Chicken and rice casserole or turkey shepherd's pie are perfect for the freezer. Just prepare the dish as usual, then cover tightly and freeze. When you're ready to eat, pop it in the oven, and dinner's served.

- Smoothie Packs: Prepare your kidney-safe smoothie *Ingredients* in advance, and store them in freezer bags. When you need a quick breakfast or snack, just blend with almond milk or water, and you're good to go!

3. Build a Meal Prep Station

One way to streamline your meal prep is to set up a "meal prep station" in your kitchen. Here's what you'll need:

- Containers: Invest in a set of reusable containers of varying sizes. These will help you portion out meals for the week. Look for BPA-free, microwave-safe, and dishwasher-safe options for convenience.
- Chopping Tools: A good set of knives, a cutting board, and a food processor can speed up your prep time. You can chop all your veggies at once, and store them in the fridge for easy access throughout the week.
- Labels and Freezer Bags: Keep labels and freezer-safe bags on hand for freezing meals. Write the date and contents on each bag to stay organized.

4. Easy One-Pot and Sheet-Pan Meals

On those days when you don't feel like prepping at all, one-pot and sheet-pan meals are your best friend. Here are a few kidney-friendly ideas:

- One-Pot Chicken and Rice: Throw some chicken, rice, and kidney-friendly veggies into one pot, add low-sodium broth, and let it cook together. Easy, balanced, and ready in under 30 minutes.
- Sheet-Pan Salmon and Veggies: Lay your salmon fillets and chopped vegetables on a baking sheet, drizzle with olive oil, and season with herbs. Pop it in the oven, and you've got a complete meal with minimal cleanup!

5. Grab-and-Go Snack Prep

Sometimes you just need something quick and healthy to snack on between meals. Prepping snacks ahead of time means you'll always have something kidney-friendly on hand. Try these easy options:

- Pre-Portioned Trail Mix: Make your own trail mix with unsalted nuts, seeds, and dried cranberries. Store them in small containers or snack bags so you can grab a handful when hunger strikes.
- Chopped Veggies and Hummus: Slice up cucumbers, bell peppers, and carrots, and pair them with low-sodium hummus. Keep them ready in your fridge for a quick and nutritious snack.

- Fruit Slices: Pre-slice apples, pears, or berries, and keep them in airtight containers. Pair with almond butter for a satisfying snack that's easy to grab and go.

Making Kidney-Supportive Habits Stick

It's one thing to know what you should be doing for your kidney health, but it's another thing entirely to make those habits stick. The truth is, forming new habits can be challenging, especially when it comes to managing CKD. But with the right approach, you can make kidney-supportive habits a regular part of your life. Here's how to turn those healthy choices into lasting routines.

1. Start Small and Be Consistent

The key to building new habits is starting small and focusing on consistency. If you try to overhaul your entire lifestyle overnight, it can feel overwhelming. Instead, focus on one or two small changes at a time. For example:

- *Start by incorporating one low-sodium meal into your day.*
- *Commit to a 10-minute walk every morning.*

- *Swap one processed snack for a kidney-friendly option like fruit or veggies with hummus.*

By setting small, achievable goals, you'll be more likely to stick with them over the long term. Once these habits become second nature, you can gradually add more.

2. Make It Enjoyable

If your new habits feel like a chore, it's unlikely they'll stick. So, find ways to make them enjoyable! For example:

- *Experiment with new kidney-friendly recipes to keep your meals exciting.*
- *Turn your walks or exercise sessions into social activities by inviting a friend or family member to join you.*
- *Treat yourself to small rewards for staying on track, like a new kitchen gadget or a cozy herbal tea.*

When you enjoy the process, it becomes much easier to stay motivated and consistent.

3. Build a Support System

Having support can make all the difference when it comes to sticking with healthy habits. Surround yourself with people who encourage your efforts and understand your goals. Here are a few ways to build a support system:

- *Share your meal planning efforts with family or friends who may also want to eat healthier.*
- *Join an online or local support group for people managing CKD. Sharing experiences and tips can be both motivating and comforting.*
- *Consider working with a dietitian or healthcare provider who specializes in CKD to help guide you in your efforts.*

The more support you have, the easier it is to stay accountable and motivated.

4. Track Your Progress

One of the most effective ways to stick to new habits is to track your progress. Seeing how far you've come can provide a great sense of accomplishment and motivate you to keep going. Here are a few things you can track:

- Meals: Keep a food diary or use a meal planning app to track your meals and see how often you're meeting your kidney-friendly goals.
- Exercise: Use a fitness app or a simple notebook to track your physical activity. Even marking off the days you go for a walk or do a yoga session can give you a sense of progress.

- Mood: Journaling about how you feel each day can help you notice any changes in your mood, energy levels, or stress levels as you adopt healthier habits.

By tracking these areas, you'll be able to see what's working and where you might need to make adjustments.

5. Be Patient with Yourself

Remember, building new habits takes time. It's normal to have days when you fall off track or feel unmotivated. The key is to be patient with yourself and not give up. If you have a bad day (or even a bad week), don't be too hard on yourself. Just pick up where you left off and keep going. Progress is progress, no matter how slow!

By following these steps, you can turn kidney-supportive habits into lifelong routines that feel natural and sustainable. Remember, it's all about finding what works for you and making small, manageable changes that add up to big improvements over time.

CHAPTER 11: BONUS PRINTABLES FOR SUCCESS

Meal Planning Printable: How to Plan Your Meals with Ease

Staying organized with your meals can feel like a challenge, but I've got you covered! This printable is designed to make meal planning a breeze. It helps you map out a week's worth of breakfast, lunch, dinner, and snacks, all while keeping your kidney health in mind.

GET THIS PRINTABLE

SCAN ME BY USING YOUR SMARTPHONE CAMERA OR A QR CODE SCANNER APP

- ✓ How to Use It: Start by writing your name at the top to make this plan truly yours. Then, for each day of the week, fill in the meal slots with recipes from this book or your own kidney-friendly favorites. Don't forget to jot down the meal times and any reminders for prepping ingredients!

- ✓ Portion Control: There's space for listing recommended portion sizes and notes from your dietitian. Use this to keep track of the portions that work best for your CKD needs.

✓ **Shopping Made Simple:** As you fill in your meals, use the shopping list area to jot down the ingredients you'll need for the week. That way, your meal plan and grocery list are all in one place.

Grocery Planning Printable: Simplifying Your Shopping

This printable takes the stress out of grocery shopping. It's split into categories—like vegetables, fruits, dairy, and proteins—so you can easily organize your trip to the store while sticking to kidney-friendly foods.

GET THIS PRINTABLE

SCAN ME BY USING YOUR SMARTPHONE CAMERA OR A QR CODE SCANNER APP

✓ **Kidney-Safe Choices:** Each category provides suggestions for foods that are lower in sodium, potassium, and phosphorus. When you're planning your grocery list, focus on these ingredients to build meals that support your health.

- ✓ Room to Customize: As you plan, fill in each section with what you need for the week. You can refer to the kidney-friendly suggestions on the side if you're not sure what to buy.
- ✓ Pro Tip: Before heading to the store, double-check your pantry for any items you already have. This helps you avoid buying unnecessary extras and stick to your meal plan.

Kidney Disease Cheat Sheet: Key Info at a Glance

This cheat sheet is your quick reference guide for eating with CKD. It lists the foods that are best for your kidneys and those you should limit or avoid. Keep this handy when planning meals or even while grocery shopping.

GET THIS PRINTABLE

SCAN ME BY USING YOUR SMARTPHONE CAMERA OR A QR CODE SCANNER APP

- ✓ Foods to Include: Use this list of kidney-friendly foods to build meals around low-potassium fruits, lean proteins, and healthy grains. It's perfect for when you need a quick reminder.

✓ Foods to Limit: The foods listed here—like red meats, high-sodium snacks, and processed foods—are ones you'll want to avoid or enjoy only in small portions. This cheat sheet helps you make healthier choices on the go.

✓ Dietary Tips: At the bottom, you'll find practical tips like how to manage portion sizes and reduce sodium. These are simple changes that can make a big difference in your CKD journey.

How to Use These Printables to Support Your Journey

These printables aren't just tools—they're part of your journey to better health. Here's how to get the most out of them:

- Meal Planning Made Easy: Use the meal planning printable to map out a week's worth of meals. It's a great way to stay on track and ensure you're getting a variety of kidney-friendly foods.

- Stress-Free Shopping: Take your grocery planning printable with you on shopping trips. By sticking to your list, you'll avoid impulse buys that might not be kidney-friendly.

- Cheat Sheet for Quick Decisions: Whether you're in the kitchen or at the store, this cheat sheet is your go-to for quick, informed decisions about what to eat.

By using these tools, you'll be able to take control of your diet and make choices that support your kidney health—one meal at a time.

---

10 Kidney-Friendly Soups for Stage 3 CKD: A Special Bonus Ebook

As a special thank you for joining me on this journey to better kidney health, I've included a bonus ebook featuring 10 carefully curated soups that are perfect for stage 3 CKD patients. These soups are not only delicious but also tailored to support your nutritional needs while helping you manage sodium, potassium, and phosphorus levels.

Why Soups? Soups are a fantastic way to enjoy nutrient-rich, kidney-friendly meals that are easy to prepare and full of flavor. Whether you're craving something light and refreshing or hearty and comforting, these soups will fit right into your weekly meal plan.

What You'll Find Inside: Each soup recipe is carefully crafted with CKD-friendly ingredients, easy-to-follow instructions, and complete nutritional information. From *Low-Sodium Chicken and Vegetable Soup to Creamy Cauliflower Soup*, these recipes are designed to make eating well as simple and enjoyable as possible.

With these soups in your cooking repertoire, you'll have a go-to resource for flavorful, kidney-friendly meals that you can enjoy all year round.

CONCLUSION

As we close this book, I want you to remember that living with stage 3 CKD is not a limitation—it's a new way of approaching your health, and I'm here with you every step of the way. Cooking and eating can still be joyful experiences, filled with flavor, variety, and balance. The recipes we've explored together are meant to support your body and nourish your spirit, giving you comfort and confidence as you manage your condition.

I often think of my dear friend Samuel, who faced his own battle with stage 3 CKD. He started his journey unsure of how he'd adapt, but through patience, persistence, and making small, kidney-friendly changes, he not only managed his condition but thrived. His determination to care for himself, one meal at a time, gave him the strength to move forward. And now, you have the tools to do the same.

The path may not always be easy, but with each recipe you make, each grocery list you prepare, you're investing in your health and your future. If Samuel could do it, so can you. Believe in the power of these small changes—they add up to something big, something life-changing.

There's a whole community out there ready to support you, from your healthcare team to others on similar journeys. Don't hesitate to reach out when you need help, guidance, or simply someone to share your experience with.

If this cookbook has made your journey a little easier, I'd love to hear from you. Your feedback helps others find their way to healthier living, just like you have. A brief review can go a long way in spreading hope and inspiration to those who need it most.

So, as you move forward, keep cooking, keep learning, and most importantly, keep believing in your ability to live well with CKD. You've got this, and I'll be with you—every step of the way.

NOTES

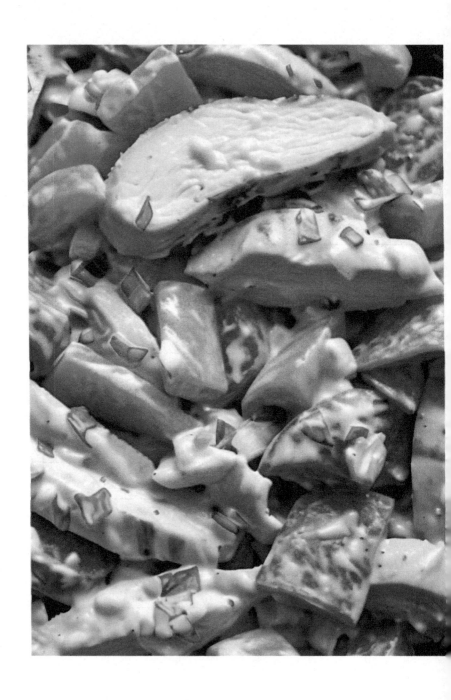

I LOOK FORWARD TO HEARING FROM YOU!

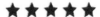

WHETHER YOU'VE JUST STARTED COOKING OR YOU'RE ALREADY ENJOYING THE RECIPES, I'D LOVE TO HEAR FROM YOU! YOUR FEEDBACK HELPS ME IMPROVE AND ALSO SUPPORTS OTHERS IN THEIR JOURNEY WITH CKD.

HOW TO LEAVE A REVIEW:

1. SCAN THE QR CODE BELOW WITH YOUR PHONE OR QR CODE SCANNER APP.
2. FOLLOW THE LINK TO THE REVIEW PAGE.
3. GIVE YOUR RATING & SHARE YOUR THOUGHTS!

EVERY REVIEW, NO MATTER HOW BRIEF, MAKES A BIG DIFFERENCE. THANK YOU SO MUCH FOR YOUR SUPPORT!

Made in United States
Orlando, FL
21 November 2024

54257673R00127